The Hippo with Toothache

Lucy H. Spelman, DVM, is the regional veterinary manager for the Mountain Gorilla Veterinary Project in central Africa, based in Rwanda. She is the former director of the Smithsonian National Zoo in Washington, D.C., and has been featured on Animal Planet and the Discovery Channel. Her website is www.drlucyspelman.com.

Ted Y. Mashima, DVM, is the president of Mashima Communication, based in Gaithersburg, Maryland. He lectures frequently and is the former associate director for the Centre for Public and Corporate Veterinary Medicine at the University of Maryland.

Praise for *The Hippo with Toothache*

'Readers will be dazzled by stories of recapturing a fugitive herd of wild bison from the outskirts of Paris and medical marvels developed to treat especially small or sensitive patients.' *Publishers Weekly*

'Some [essays] end in sorrow, most have happy endings. What comes across in each is the love, respect, and dedication vets have for their patients. Definitely recommended.' *ScienceBlogs*

'The ongoing popularity of veterinary memoirs makes this a worthy purchase, and the episodic nature of the individual stories makes it a perfect book for dipping into.' *Booklist*

'A stunning array of stories from twenty-eight of the best wild animal veterinarians in all parts of the world . . . [They] are contributing indispensable knowledge to a worldwide effort to protect wild creatures threatened by human activity. My hat is off to these unsung heroes of the natural world.' Roger Sant, chair of the Board of Regents, Smithsonian Institution

'This is a delightful book. The stories, each amazingly different, are told with warmth, humor, and sensitivity. They are sometimes sad, always captivating. It is a book you can dip into on a journey or read before sleep at night. Buy it and give copies to your friends.' Dr. Jane Goodall, DBE, founder, the Jane Goodall Institute; UN Messenger of Peace

'Spelman and Mashima's fascinating exploration of the mysterious and often exciting world of veterinary medicine within the confines of the zoological community is a rare opportunity for the reader to go behind the scenes, where the stories of drama, discovery, and compassion have been waiting to be revealed. This book is a compelling journey of the often herculean efforts on behalf of dedicated zoo veterinarians and their charismatic patients. . . . It is a journey of triumph and tragedy, mystery and discovery, which will keep the reader glued to the pages like the prosthetic shoes glued to a rhino hoof.' Jeff Corwin, wildlife biologist and television presenter for *Animal Planet* and Discovery networks

'This is an inspiring collection of true stories written with respect and affection for wild animals.' Jim Maddy, president & CEO, Association of Zoos and Aquariums

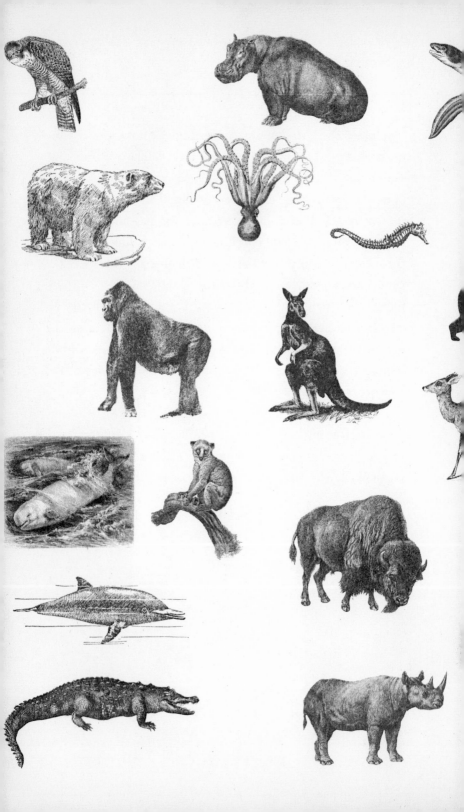

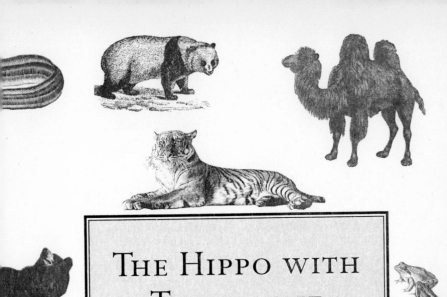

The Hippo with Toothache

Heart-warming Stories of Zoo and Wild Animals and the Vets who Care for Them

Edited by

Lucy H. Spelman, DVM

and

Ted Y. Mashima, DVM

Foreword by Jack Hanna

rh
BOOKS

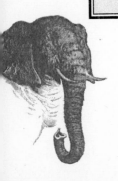
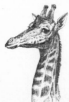

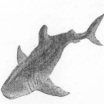

Published by Random House Books 2009

4 6 8 10 9 7 5 3

Copyright Lucy H. Spelman and Ted Y. Mashima © 2009

Lucy H. Spelman amd Ted Y Mashima have asserted their right under the Copyright, Designs and Patents Act, 1988, to be identified as the authors of this work

First published in the United States as *The Rhino with Glue-on Shoes* by Delacorte Press, an imprint of The Random House Publishing Group, a division of Random House Inc. in 2008

First published in Great Britain in 2009 by
Random House Books
Random House, 20 Vauxhall Bridge Road,
London SW1V 2SA

www.rbooks.co.uk

Addresses for companies within The Random House Group Limited can be found at:
www.randomhouse.co.uk/offices.htm

The Random House Group Limited Reg. No. 954009

A CIP catalogue record for this book
is available from the British Library

ISBN 9781847945983

Penguin Random House is committed to a sustainable future for our business, our readers and our planet. This book is made from Forest Stewardship Council® certified paper.

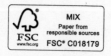

Printed and bound in Great Britain by Clays Ltd, Elcograf S.p.A.

Text design by Glen M. Edelstein

For
Mary Lockwood Spelman
and
Edward Kozo Mashima

Contents

Foreword

by Jack Hanna

Patient. Persevering. Caring. Compassionate. Dedicated. Highly-skilled and ingenious. These are just a few of the words that describe veterinarians, people who have basically given their lives over to the well-being of our animal friends.

During thirty-plus years working with all kinds of creatures, I've met many vets around the world. Whether they treat our family pets or take care of wild animals in zoos or in remote locations, these doctors are made from the same exceptional mold.

Veterinarians can't meet friends for dinner on a Saturday night without the possibility of being called away to treat an ailing critter. There's no such thing as an average day at the office. Emergencies happen daily—and without warning. Some animals are treated quickly, while others take days, weeks, and even months of treatment. If there's no progress, vets go to work exploring other avenues to get their patients back on their own four (or two) feet.

In diagnosing patients who cannot talk and don't understand what is being done to them, vets have to be extremely resourceful and creative, and those doctors who work with wild animals even more so. What do you do with an eel that won't eat, for example? Or with an animal in the forest that you know is injured, but you can't even find. Some animals manage to hide from the doctor for days or even weeks. In these cases, it takes a combination of stamina, smarts, intuition, and a bit of luck just to find the patient—and that's not even the hardest part. How do you pacify a creature to whom you are entirely alien? How do you, for instance, help calm the nerves of a whale shark riding in a huge fish tank perched on a ship that is pitching up and down on a rolling sea?

Vets encounter such troubles every day, and must deal with them with a clear head and psychological detachment. That's a tough job! Often, these doctors can't separate themselves completely. They too must endure worry and sadness. Vets' lives are intertwined with their animal patients. Those of us who work with wild animals develop bonds with them as well—usually from a safe distance, of course. The special relationship we have with a favorite animal, whether it's an octopus or a tiger, makes it hard for us to see it suffer in any way.

Every animal can benefit from veterinary care. This field of science has come a long way in recent times, and wild animals—here at home and around the globe—have benefited tremendously. Technology has made diagnosis and treatment much better and more efficient. Vets now treat wild animals in zoos, aquaria, national parks, and wildlife reserves, paving the way for greater successes in conservation. These doctors help breeding groups of endangered species live longer and healthier reproductive lives, often using sophisticated techniques to help them reproduce more quickly. They also treat wild animals in their natural habitats.

In Lucy Spelman and Ted Mashima's wonderful and inspiring book, *The Rhino with Glue-On Shoes*, you'll discover what it's like to be a vet working with wild animals in every imaginable setting. Through this collection of tales told by vets from around the globe, you'll explore their odd, interesting, sometimes crazy world, and enjoy every minute.

These stories demonstrate what zoo, aquaria, and wild animal veterinarians are made of. They are tough and resilient people, highly trained doctors, caring souls who have dedicated their lives here on Earth to the animals we love. In the process, they develop a "oneness" with animals. I like to think this is true for all of us. From the funny Texas dung beetles to the majestic African elephant, we are a part of Earth's life forms and thus share a common bond.

At one time, such work with endangered animals was only a dream. I hope that veterinary care for both captive- and free-living wild animals continues to increase. Sadly, there are many small, isolated populations of rare species worldwide that need help from each and every one of us. If we respect all creatures, as the vets in this book do, we can help maintain nature's delicate balance.

Jack Hanna
Director Emeritus, Columbus Zoo
Host, TV's *Jack Hanna's Into the Wild*

Introduction

As zoo vets, we are often asked to share our true stories, our most memorable cases. We lecture, visit schools, attend fund-raisers, lead behind-the-scenes tours, write for newsletters, and give interviews to the media. We usually begin by explaining that virtually anything is possible in our profession: intensive care for a turtle with a crushed shell, ultrasound to confirm pregnancy in a dolphin, cataract removal in an eagle.

The title "zoo vet" is expandable to "zoo and wildlife vet," "wild animal vet," and "aquatic vet." Each refers to the same basic profession, the practice of zoological medicine, defined as medical care for wild animals as opposed to domestic ones. These veterinarians work for zoos, aquaria, universities, wildlife rehabilitation centers, national parks, and protected wilderness areas. They also contribute their expertise on behalf of conservation and endangered species.

So what's it like to be a zoo vet? people often ask. How close do you get to your patients? Have you ever been injured by one of them? Do you become attached to the animals, and if so, isn't it hard when they die?

Some questions touch on the ethics of keeping or confining wild animals: Don't you wish all of your patients could live freely? Conversely, is anything truly "wild" anymore?

We hope the stories in this book, written by twenty-nine of today's top zoo vets, will answer many of these questions— and others the reader may not even have thought of. Our contributing authors bring unique perspectives to each case, depending on their training, the settings in which they work, and the motivation that inspired them to become vets in the first place. Their exotic and interesting patients range all over the animal kingdom, including a rhino with chronic foot problems, an orphaned whale calf, a kangaroo with a broken neck, a herd of escaped bison, and an anorexic eel.

Though every case is different in this compilation, certain patterns emerge. The big challenge for any zoo vet is to distinguish the normal from the abnormal. In the process, we tackle the same set of problems: when, where, and how to get our hands on the animal, and what—if anything—to do for it. Since our patients don't walk into the clinic on the end of a leash, even a simple physical exam requires some type of restraint or anesthesia. To avoid the associated risk, zoo vets usually observe first and act second.

Wild animals are also exceptionally good at hiding clinical signs of injury or illness, aside from the obvious broken limb or squirting diarrhea. Their doctors look for subtle changes in attitude, activity, or appetite. In response, the patient learns to accept the watchful gaze of any human who carries a stethoscope, wears binoculars, or smells faintly of disinfectant.

Once the diagnosis is made and treatment begins, vets rely

even more on their nontechnical skills. Like Dr. Dolittle, they know the most reliable information comes from the animal itself, and they'll frequently check in on their patients. Compassion, empathy, and a bit of intuition go a long way toward helping wild animals heal.

We offer these stories not only to illustrate the complexity of modern zoological medicine but also to give the general reader a rare opportunity to experience the special bonds that develop between zoo vets and their wild animal patients.

Lucy H. Spelman, DVM, and Ted Y. Mashima, DVM

THE HIPPO WITH
TOOTHACHE

I

CLOSE CONNECTIONS

Pediatricians who work with infants and vets who work with wild animals share a major challenge: their patients can't speak. Each must rely on someone else to tell them what's wrong. The physician asks the child's parent several all-important questions: When did this start? What are the symptoms? Is the patient better or worse today? Domestic animal vets ask the same questions of the pet owner or farmer. But zoo vets must seek out this information from a variety of keepers, animal caretakers, curators, managers, and scientists, and it may often be sketchy or incomplete.

After gathering bits and pieces of history, our next step is to observe the animal. Unfortunately, most of our patients either run away or threaten resistance when they see the vet coming. Hooved animals, birds, and reptiles will flee if they can; tigers, bears, Komodo dragons, and other predators may show aggression. We can easily pick up tiny animals like frogs and jellyfish, but handling them has been shown to cause them stress. So our first exam is a visual one, performed from a safe distance, often with a good set of binoculars.

It's at this point that we develop an initial bond with the patient. The wild animal begins to tolerate our presence. In cases where the injury or illness is mild, that may be the extent of our interaction. But if we need more information, the relationship intensifies. In order to treat untamed animals, zoo vets must find ways to connect with their patients—without being bitten, scratched, kicked, or poisoned.

Some wild animals can be conditioned to the presence, and even the touch, of a doctor. In exchange for a food treat, zoo rhinos will stand quietly in a stall for ultrasound examination. Free-living mountain gorillas will allow vets to approach within a few feet to observe a wound. But with most wild animal patients, the only way to gather the necessary health data is to capture and anesthetize them for a complete exam.

Now our connection to the animal becomes much more tangible. A hands-on exam offers an invaluable opportunity to examine an individual thoroughly. It may even serve as our first introduction to a species. In the backs of our minds, we're curious about, even in awe of, our patients. So we work in teams of vets and technicians in order to learn as much as possible in a short amount of time. While we focus on the health problem at hand, we also document the normal anatomy and take samples to establish baseline physiological data.

If the animal is chronically ill, requiring repeat exams, the relationship between doctor and patient becomes more dynamic. Tolerance develops into familiarity, mutual respect, even companionship. This is particularly true with highly intelligent and long-lived species like great apes, elephants, dolphins, whales, tortoises, parrots, and raptors. And always there is the bond of responsibility: each veterinarian takes a professional oath to help animals in need.

Emotions can also fuel and shape these bonds. We feel anxiety about the best course of treatment, relief when the patient recovers, sadness if it dies. For difficult and unusual cases, we rack our brains, pore through textbooks and journals, and call our colleagues for advice. After four hours of surgery on a polar bear or a nightlong vigil with a kangaroo in intensive care, we worry about the outcome. We put all of our veterinary skills on the line.

If the patient recovers, we're happy for the animal, professionally satisfied, and personally relieved. More often than not, however, the animal feels the exact opposite about us. Every zoo vet has a story about a former patient that thanks its doctor by hissing or spitting, throwing excrement, or roaring and charging.

Inevitably, there are cases where we fail. The diagnosis may elude us, the injury may be too severe, or advanced medical therapy may not be practical or possible for a wild animal. In such situations, our job is to alleviate suffering, which sometimes includes euthanasia. Our relationship with the animal helps us make such decisions with compassion, empathy, and concern for the animal's quality of life.

In the stories that follow, doctor and patient form especially close connections. Each bond is unique, and some are closer and more emotional than others. The patients include an eel, a chimpanzee, a fawn, a bear cub, and a whale calf.

Lucy H. Spelman, DVM

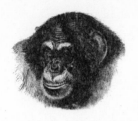

Tough Guy Hondo

by Barb Wolfe, DVM, PhD

Chimps are a disgusting, violent society," advised my colleague as I contemplated the group of thirteen in front of me. This was early in my career, and as the new veterinarian at the North Carolina Zoo in 1997, I didn't know much about chimpanzee behavior. I stood watching the peaceable group in silent disagreement. A two-year-old wobbled by with a towel on her head. Two juveniles were donning socks for fun, while others poked at bits of food with sticks or bulldozed piles of straw around in circles with their lanky arms. I was marveling at my good fortune. I had a great job—and my first task of the day was to meet the chimp keepers and learn about these amusing animals in their care.

Punctuating that thought, a low howl began in the room, growing rapidly into a crescendo of hoots and screams. The keeper beside me said softly, "Just hold still." I searched the group for the source of the noise. Hondo, the dominant male, was looking directly at me, bobbing up and down menacingly, while the rest of the group darted frantically about whooping the equivalent of a chimp-language emergency signal. Suddenly, Hondo bounded from the back of the enclosure, launched himself onto the mesh between us, and spat what felt like an ocean of water in my face. I didn't hold still. I reeled involuntarily backward, stumbled on a pile of hoses, and ended up propped against a wall—soaked, horrified, embarrassed, and not entirely sure that I couldn't catch Ebola virus from captive chimp spit.

It had never occurred to me that zoo animals would resent their vets. We are hardwired to love animals. We spend our whole lives plotting this career, scooping up clinic poop as kids, getting good grades even in the classes we hate, and volunteering our way through life long beyond the time when our childhood friends are having kids and buying houses. All to get to this glorious station: Zoo Vet. Then we find out that most animals can smell a vet coming before the truck rattles into the driveway, and will prepare their most unwelcoming demeanor. If they have limbs capable of hurling something, they will find something to hurl. If they can emit a nasty smell, they will be at their smelliest when you get there. And those with teeth and loud voices? Well, despite the thickest steel bars between you, being four feet from a lion that has just received a dart and is standing full height and roaring at you can truly necessitate a wardrobe change.

Hondo was no exception, and he greeted me the same way every time I paid the chimps a visit during those first few years. The way to cure him, the keepers said, was to ignore the assault. Just the way we tell our kids to deal with bullies. So year after year, every time a chimp had a runny nose or a cut on its finger, I would approach the enclosure calmly and try to examine the patient with composure while the keeper rewarded it with fruit juice or yogurt through the mesh. Out of the corner of my eye, I would see Hondo filling his mouth at the water spigot. Then, inevitably, the warning hoots of the troop would begin, the patient would dart fearfully away, and Hondo would appear, like a flying King Kong, to give me a dousing. I'd quietly stand up, dripping spit from my eyelashes, issue suggestions for treatment of the patient, and retreat without even the solace of a threatening glare at him.

Reportedly, a previous vet used to wear bright yellow rain gear to protect himself when entering the chimp building. Hondo was delighted to see this costume change on his behalf, and ramped up the ferocity of his attack. He wasn't like Joey, the sneaky sea lion who would bite you when you weren't paying attention. You could stare Joey into submission, the way a border collie does with sheep. Making eye contact with Hondo only accelerated the strike. There was nothing I could do, and I began to regard him as the enemy.

The vets weren't his only target, though. Hondo also had a habit of throwing rocks at visitors from his grassy knoll in the center of the chimp enclosure. The zoo had to build an entirely new exhibit to protect the public from Hondo's expressions of hospitality.

The new habitat that emerged amounted to an expansive chimpanzee resort, furnished with a thirty-foot-high climbing tree, hammocks, plenty of natural vegetation, logs for climbing, and even a fake African termite mound. Zoo visitors enjoyed a clear, close view of the animals, protected by fifteen-foot walls of thick rock-proof, spit-proof glass. You could walk right up to the chimps, who stood on the same level, crouch in front of them, look them in the eye, and even "touch" them by pressing your hand against the glass where they offered theirs. From the way the chimps flocked to the glass to view people up close, they were equally impressed. And on opening day, with a large group of VIPs attending the ribbon-cutting ceremony, Hondo celebrated by lobbing a square-foot slab of rock up and over the new glass wall at the crowd.

But as time went on, the new exhibit seemed to temper Hondo's animosity. On one visit, I bent down to indulge Jonathan, a homely youngster with car-door ears, who was pressing his face against the glass as if to kiss me. I saw Hondo tanking up at the spigot in the background, and started to steel myself for the deluge before I realized I was safe. Instead of submissively averting my gaze, I looked him in the eye. Hondo ambled up and sat in front of me, and we regarded each other coolly. He'd swallowed his mouthful of water—maybe experience had taught him that the glass, if not the vet, spits back. He just sat and watched me intently for a minute, then began alternately touching his bottom lip and then his chest, as if to say "Me" or "Feed me." I mimicked him, and he repeated the sequence back to me. I asked the keepers what this behavior meant, but no one knew. He just did that sometimes.

From time to time thereafter, when I went to the chimp building, I'd wander out to the exhibit first. Hondo often greeted me at the glass, sitting quietly in front of me and sometimes playing our version of charades. The visitors would all gather around excitedly and ask questions about what he was saying to me. I figured anything he really had to say to me probably couldn't be repeated, but smiled inwardly at the idea that they might harbor a belief that zoo vets were real-life Dr. Dolittles and could simply "ask" the animals what was wrong with them. The truth is sometimes we wish we had a crystal ball.

One day, the keepers noted that Hondo had taken on a new habit: head-standing. I went to the exhibit and he came over to the glass for a visit. Rather than sit with me, though, he stood up and pressed the top of his head onto the grass as if looking backward between his legs. He kept this up for several minutes, stopping only to look up and see if anyone was still watching him. There are two primary causes of head-pressing in animals: head pain and liver disease. Knowing that Hondo had a cataract in one eye, we wondered if he might be developing glaucoma, a painful buildup of pressure within the eyeball.

Our consulting veterinary ophthalmologist kindly offered to donate his time for this interesting case, and we anesthetized Hondo for a complete examination. The general exam checked out well, but the ophthalmologic exam confirmed our suspicion: the long-standing cataract had caused severe, untreatable glaucoma, and the eye needed to be removed. After the diagnostic procedure, the ophthalmologist offered two options. We could remove the inner workings of the eye, leaving the outer shell in place and filling the space with a silicone rubber-ball prosthesis, or we could give him a false eye prosthesis used in human medicine—the kind that can be taken out and popped back in at will.

I looked up at this quiet, knowledgeable eye doctor and wondered why a veterinary ophthalmologist would ever offer the latter option. Ophthalmologists routinely perform amazing procedures that restore function to this complicated organ, but there are some tools in their tool belt that simply aren't practical in the animal world. They know so much about the eye, in fact, that they can identify a species by looking at the retina, inside the eye. We had to learn this skill in vet school ophthalmology class, as if at some point in our veterinary career we might come across an eyeball—rolling around on the ground, for instance—that needed to be treated and wasn't currently attached to the species to which it belonged. I momentarily contemplated the hours spent rummaging through the bushes to find the fake eyeball every time Hondo yanked it out to throw it at someone, and opted for the stay-in-the-socket prosthesis.

The surgery went well, and Hondo's head-standing ceased immediately. His postsurgical care, however, required daily visual exams and eyedrops. I visited him often in his holding area, where, eyeball-to-eyeball, I could check the surgery site and take follow-up photos without the intervening glass. One day, with little more than the expensive camera equipment between us, I realized that he had stopped spitting water on me. How could that be? After all the years of spitting when I was careful not to even look at him, the recent weeks of anesthetic darts, surgery, frequent exams, antibiotic treatments, and eyedrops had somehow improved our relationship. Not only that, Hondo readily approached to sit with me, giving up the opportunity to impress the chimp troop by humiliating me with a mouthful of water.

On one visit, when Hondo's recovery was nearly complete, he began another new ritual. He reached his index finger through the mesh, as if asking to touch my gloved finger. When I finally mustered the courage to allow him to touch the very tip of my finger, he held it there, staring at it, as if fascinated by my latex skin.

The keepers started making jokes about our relationship, asking me to visit him even when he didn't need a vet check. Hondo had a well-known fondness for certain women, and now, apparently, I was one of them. I secretly relished the fact that here was a zoo animal that might just like me. When chimpanzee annual physical exams came around every year, I made sure I wasn't the one to shoot Hondo with the dart gun. The chimps take this very personally, and are masters of dart evasion. Once you've withstood the screaming, lunging, fecal projectiles, and wall-beating long enough to deliver an accurate shot, you have to move quickly in case the chimp decides to throw the dart back at you. I've seen one dramatic female pull her dart out, approach the wire mesh, vocalizing pathetically, sit down, squeeze the tiny hole in her thigh, touch it with her finger, and show the drop of blood to her keeper, drawing coos of sympathy before she fell asleep. I didn't want Hondo to associate me with this indignity, so I stayed out of sight until he was asleep.

One year, during Hondo's physical exam, I felt a lump. It was a large, very firm area of his liver near his rib cage. I swallowed hard, prepped him for minor surgery, and took a needle biopsy of his liver through the skin. A few days later, with the pathologists' report in hand, I had the dismal job of talking to the keepers about Hondo's diagnosis. It's hard to imagine the level of emotion that develops between keepers and these intelligent, sentient close relatives of ours. My bond with him was special, but I bounced around the zoo every day treating hundreds of different mammals, birds, reptiles, and fish. His keepers spent every daylight hour with the chimp troop, training, feeding, cleaning, and communicating with them. They were family.

I explained to the somber group that Hondo had hepatic amyloidosis, an accumulation of inflammatory protein in the liver. The cause was unknown, and there was no specific treatment for it. The only thing we could reasonably do to help him would be to keep him out of fights—a natural part of chimp culture—because the liver was involved with blood clotting. He could bleed to death from a serious bite wound.

The keepers and curators decided to separate Hondo from the unruly female chimps, so he could lead a quiet life with Jonathan, the homely and mischievous young male. There was no way to know how long Hondo would live. At the request of the teary-eyed keepers, I visited him in his holding area, and was heartbroken to find him lying on his back, looking weak and in obvious pain. When he saw me, he reached his index finger through the mesh. I offered mine, and he stroked my finger slowly. I felt powerless.

But Hondo didn't. Being retired from the difficult job of keeping ten cranky, argumentative female apes in line agreed with him immediately. He and Jonathan spent their days swinging from fire hoses, eating giant lettuce leaves, throwing dirt, wearing their play socks, and basking in the sun in their enormous exhibit. Hondo gained weight, grew more hair, and looked healthier than ever. A year later, he was reintroduced to the troop, and regained control of his females. He remains that way today. He's not cured, but perhaps the time away from the troop reduced the stressors in his life, making it easier for his body to fight the liver disease.

I've been away from the zoo for nearly two years now, and I miss Hondo and his comrades. When I have the chance to visit, I head straight for the chimp exhibit. He still gets quiet and comes over to have a chat with me. I know he misses me too—because, well, he did spit on the new veterinarian.

ABOUT THE AUTHOR

Barbara Wolfe grew up in Cincinnati, Ohio, and avidly read animal behavior books as a child. She received her bachelor of science degree in molecular genetics from the University of California, Davis, and her veterinary degree followed by a PhD in reproductive physiology from Texas A&M University. Dr. Wolfe's interest in zoo medicine began with her research in assisted reproduction of endangered species, which has ranged from antelope to cats to elephants. Board certified by the American College of Zoological Medicine, she has worked as a researcher and veterinarian for the National Zoo and the North Carolina Zoo, and is currently the director of wildlife and conservation medicine at the Wilds in Cumberland, Ohio. She is an associate editor for the *Journal of Zoo and Wildlife Medicine*, serves on the Wildlife Scientific Advisory Board for the Morris Animal Foundation, and still finds animal behavior fascinating.

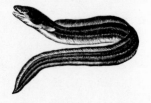

The Eel and the Bartender

by Beth Chittick Nolan, DVM, MS

A green moray eel was donated to the New England
Aquarium by a bartender from a neighboring state. For
years, the eel had lived in a tank next to the bar, but it had begun to outgrow its home.

In the wild, green morays are found in warm marine habitats such as rocky shorelines and coral reefs. They are solitary
fish, spending most of the day hidden in crevices and emerging at night to hunt fish, shrimp, crabs, or cephalopods. From
what I could gather, this eel was no shrinking violet. It had
been a favorite among patrons, who would regularly check
on it during their bar visits.

When the eel first arrived at the aquarium in the late
1990s, we set up a large holding tank along a back wall of
the gallery. There it was quarantined from other fish in the

collection until we were sure it was healthy and doing well in its new environment. Soon after its arrival, it settled in behind the rockwork of the tank, as eels often do.

For the first several days, the eel hid in its nook and refused food. This is not uncommon for some fish, especially after a move. The days lengthened to a week, and then to two weeks. The eel stayed hidden and would not emerge to eat.

It had come to us with very little history about its eating habits. The diet must have been fairly balanced, considering it had already grown to nearly three feet in length—or roughly half adult size. Maybe someone periodically tossed it a couple of chicken wings.

With aquatic animals, ensuring good housing, water quality, and nutrition is critical to keeping them healthy. Some robust eels can fast for many days, even for a couple of weeks after a major environmental change. With longer fasting periods, though, the eel's general health could become compromised.

The aquarists started trying all of the tricks of the trade to get this eel to eat. They enticed it with a variety of foods of different sizes, shapes, and flavors. They tried chopped capelin and herring, whole shrimp and pieces of squid, even live bait, but the eel showed no interest. The water quality was constantly monitored to ensure all parameters were within the preferred ranges for eels. The aquarists even tried covering the tank and dimming the lights to reduce stress to the eel and, some of them joked, "to simulate the eel's previous dark barlike ambience." But all the efforts were to no avail. The moray refused to eat.

In the third week, the aquarists were growing more concerned and I got more involved. Could the eel's lack of appetite be related to a medical problem? We discussed diagnostic options, including blood work and parasite screening, as well as possible treatments such as tube feeding. We decided to examine the patient, which requires sedation in eels unless one is particularly proficient at holding on to a slippery, mucus-coated, snakelike animal with sharp teeth.

We netted the eel and transferred it to a covered bucket of tank water with dissolved anesthetic powder. An air stone bubbled in the water to keep it adequately oxygenated during the procedure. The first signs of sedation became evident as the eel's gilling rate slowed and it began to lie on its side. Within a few minutes, it was relaxed enough to be held safely out of the water without it struggling.

I thoroughly examined the moray, checking for any evidence of health problems. Its pale green skin was coated with a thin layer of mucus, which is as expected for these animals. I didn't see any fraying or irregularities in its long ribbonlike dorsal fin or tail. Its abdomen did not appear to be distended or otherwise abnormal. Its gills were a normal deep red and its mouth, with all of its teeth, looked fine. As with any routine fish workup, I collected a small sample of gill tissue and feces, as well as a scraping of skin mucus, to evaluate under the microscope for parasites, but saw none. I took a blood sample from its tail vein, but the results showed no abnormalities—no elevated white count or anything else that would suggest illness.

After collecting our diagnostic samples, we passed a small rubber tube through the eel's mouth into its stomach and injected some fish gruel. At least we could give it some nutrition that day. Then we placed it back in its tank, syringing salt water over its gills to reverse the sedation. Within a few minutes, it started to swim on its own. Before long, it settled right back into its hiding spot behind the rockwork.

As I sat there worrying about this eel, I found myself remembering the more mundane roles fish played in my childhood. My earliest experiences with fish were probably eating fish sticks, those processed finger-food wonders. During my elementary school days, fish were the small minnows my brother and I scampered through creeks to catch. When I was a bit older, fish were the three-inch sunnies we'd proudly display for the camera when fishing with Dad. Fish were the prey of gulls and gruff-looking old men casting off the jetties of Long Island Sound.

In fifth grade, I won Small Fry at the school fair, much to my delight and my mother's chagrin. Although I liked my pet goldfish, and would watch him in his small bowl, I was sad but not crushed when he met an untimely death (Mom deloused the house one afternoon and unfortunately deloused Small Fry as well). After all, it was "just a fish," as someone had told me.

So I certainly had no childhood aspirations to become a fish doctor. During my fourth year in veterinary school, however, I got the opportunity to shadow the head vet at the New England Aquarium for a month. To my surprise, I was fascinated by the daily challenges and discoveries of aquatic animal medicine, a field that few veterinarians venture to tackle because it includes a great many species about which we know relatively little. From invertebrate animals like jellyfish and lobsters to vertebrates such as fish, sea turtles, and marine mammals, aquatic medicine covers a wide diversity of animals that receive minimal, if any, attention in the standard veterinary school curricula.

Just a couple years later, here I was, the intern veterinarian at the aquarium, now faced with an anorexic moray eel.

The question remained: Why was this animal refusing to eat? After three weeks, wasn't he hungry? We could support it nutritionally with tube feeding, but for how long? We were all stumped by the case.

Finally, one of the aquarists suggested that we contact the bartender who'd donated the eel. Maybe he would give us some ideas to stimulate this eel's appetite. Although less than optimistic about the outcome, we had few other alternatives and needed this poor eel to eat. We made the call.

After hearing the news and failing to come up with any immediate suggestions on how to better feed the eel, the bartender offered to pay it a visit. I happened to be in the gallery by the eel tank when a large, broad-shouldered man entered one morning. The bartender approached the tank somewhat apprehensively, a furrowed brow shadowing his features. He quietly stood in front of the tank—and waited.

At the bottom edge of the rockwork, in the far corner of the tank, a small head appeared. It hesitated, surveying its surroundings, and then slowly, ever so slowly, pulled its lean body from its lair. It cautiously moved directly in front of the man. The eel paused. Its round lidless eyes focused intently on the man's face. Then, to my amazement, the eel began to undulate its body back and forth in a smooth, calm rhythm, maintaining eye contact with the man the entire time. The man's worried look softened as the corners of his mouth lifted. Here was his old friend again.

I don't remember the words of endearment the man said that day. I remember that the man hand-fed the eel a piece of fish or shrimp, and that the eel did not refuse food from that day forward. But most of all, I remember the look of pure adoration on the man's face as this eel emerged from its hiding place for him, and only him.

I have experienced the strength and love of the human-animal bond many times since then over the years. In practice, I have witnessed many clients with close bonds to their pets, large and small, furred and feathered. But despite all my veterinary training, my growing fascination with sea creatures, and my own personal experience, I had never truly considered the potential for such a close connection between man and fish until that eel and bartender taught me otherwise. Their bond was even more elemental than the eel's hunger for food.

ABOUT THE AUTHOR

Born and raised in Connecticut, Elizabeth Chittick Nolan dreamed initially of becoming a field biologist in the wilds of Africa but set her sights on veterinary medicine while at Haverford College. After earning her biology degree, she attended Tufts University School of Veterinary Medicine. In her fourth year, a monthlong rotation at New England Aquarium piqued her interest in aquatic medicine. Dr. Nolan completed two internships in Boston, one in small animal medicine and surgery at the Angell Memorial Animal Hospital, the second in aquatic animal medicine at New England Aquarium. To specialize further in nondomestic animals, she accepted a zoological medicine residency at

North Carolina State University and later became board certified through the American College of Zoological Medicine. She spent the next five years as a staff veterinarian at SeaWorld Orlando, where she gained valuable experience in the aquatic animal field. In 2006, Dr. Nolan decided to broaden her horizons again by accepting a veterinary position with Disney's Animal Programs—"a job I'm thoroughly enjoying!"

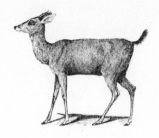

Earring Boy

by Ned Gentz, DVM

It was summer 1997, a hot, humid July day in Virginia's Shenandoah Valley. The van with the out-of-state license plates in the parking lot of a grocery store in Harrisonburg had its windows rolled up tight. Two concerned good Samaritans, studying the van, saw someone or something moving inside—a child, perhaps, or a pet. They called the police. When the van's owners emerged from the grocery store, they were surprised to find their car staked out by two of Harrisonburg's finest. Then it was the officers' turn to be surprised as the two women, a mother and daughter, unlocked and opened the van: inside was a young male white-tailed deer fawn. The policemen summoned a state game warden and began gathering information.

The younger of the two women told the police she'd been

driving her mother from North Carolina to Virginia for a visit to her home in Harrisonburg five days earlier when they came upon the spotted fawn. It was lying in the grass alongside the road near Roanoke, Virginia. The fawn's mother had been struck and killed by a car, she said. Not knowing what else to do, she added, they'd picked up the little Bambi, put him in the back of their van, and kept driving. They'd kept the animal with them ever since.

When the police checked the back of the van, they found the spotted fawn panting heavily from the heat. It was wearing a disposable diaper because it had developed scours (diarrhea) from the cow's milk the women had given him. Even more bizarrely, the bright sunshine streaming in through the van's open door glittered as it struck the little fawn's ears. The police stared at the animal in disbelief. Each ear was pierced with a cross-shaped rhinestone earring.

The game warden arrived and announced that he was confiscating the fawn, to the histrionic objections of the two women. He placed a call to the Wildlife Center of Virginia (WCV) in Waynesboro, where I was the head veterinarian. The WCV is a wildlife hospital and wildlife education center that routinely cares for several thousand sick, injured, and orphaned wild animals each year. Of course, we told the game warden, we'd be glad to check out the fawn and make sure it was okay.

When the fawn arrived, I performed a physical examination. My trusty hospital manager and head veterinary technician, Sarah Snead, restrained and calmed the nervous youngster. He weighed just thirteen pounds, and we guessed him to be only a few weeks old. There was no way we could release this baby into the wild. I'd have to hold the fawn in our facility for several months until he was old enough to fend for himself.

The fawn was dehydrated from the combination of heat and diarrhea. He also had an elevated temperature from being confined in the hot van. I removed the earrings from the fawn's ears. Both ears were infected: the skin around the holes was red and inflamed.

I treated the fawn's dehydration with subcutaneous fluids, injected under the skin in several places across his back. The animal would gradually absorb the liquid. Once it was gone, we'd repeat the treatment several times. Then I started the fawn on antibiotic therapy—injections of penicillin—for the ear infections. I also treated these with a topical antibiotic.

Next we had to deal with the scours and the presumptive tummyache that went along with them. Since fawn season had recently begun in western Virginia, we'd already received an initial supply of goat's milk in preparation for the orphaned white-tailed deer fawns we knew would be coming our way.

From prior experience, we knew that either fresh goat's milk or powdered lamb-milk replacer worked best for raising orphan deer fawns; cow's milk is not so good. The trick is not to overload the digestive system too fast, especially in a dehydrated animal. The fawn's first bottle would be 25 percent goat's milk and 75 percent water, the second one 50-50, and the third 75 percent goat's milk and 25 percent water. That way, we'd allow the animal's intestinal tract time to adjust before starting on pure goat's milk. Our new fawn was hungry and took to the bottle readily. The holes in his ears healed in about two weeks, and I discontinued the antibiotics.

The WCV routinely receives twenty to thirty white-tailed deer fawns every year. Some of these fawns are legitimately orphaned, found standing next to their dead mothers alongside a roadway after a fatal encounter with a car that couldn't stop in time. But many "orphaned" fawns aren't orphaned at all. Mother deer don't spend all day with their babies. On the contrary, they allow the fawns to nurse only a few times a day. Most of the time, deer moms are out shopping for groceries (as it were) while they leave their babies hidden in a nest of tall grass somewhere. A fawn has the instinct to lie very still, not moving until it hears its mother coming back for it.

Unfortunately, most people who happen upon such a fawn in a field or woods think the baby has been abandoned. It's all too easy for them to pick up the animal and carry it away, thinking they are doing the right thing for the fawn. But taking a perfectly healthy animal out of the wild is obviously not in its best interest.

Whenever a new orphan arrived, I'd quiz its would-be rescuers, trying to ascertain whether they'd actually seen a dead mom. If not, I'd encourage them to put the fawn back where they found it.

Some people worry that "the scent of man" carried by such a fawn will deter the mother from taking her baby back. But this is rarely the case. Of course, a replaced baby does need to be monitored to make sure its mother returns to care for it. Most of the time, putting these babies back where they came from works. Was our new fawn with the rhinestone earrings a true orphan or not? From the vague story told by his female captors, I feared we'd never know for sure.

Happily, he already had a companion. We'd recently received our first orphan deer fawn of the year—good timing for Earring Boy, as my wildlife rehabilitation staff had taken to calling him. We didn't routinely give names to the wild animals in our care at the WCV. We wanted to stress that these animals were not pets, that our goal was to make them better and then return them to the wild. More important, deer fawns are best raised in groups and with minimal contact with people, so that they retain their wild instincts. Nevertheless the name stuck.

When the game wardens called to check on Earring Boy, I told them he was doing fine. Good, they replied, because we need you to keep him there until the court date. They were charging the women in the van with illegal possession of wildlife: you can't go driving around with a live deer in the back of your car. Because of the earrings, the women would also be charged with cruelty to a wild animal. I would have to go to court as a potential witness when the case was heard before the judge.

In an odd sort of way, I looked forward to the court date. It wasn't just that I didn't think Earring Boy was a true orphan. I believed it was important to address the all-too-common problem of people taking wild animals out of the wild. Without seeking expert advice, people will often keep a wild animal for a few days, thinking it will make a good pet, until it becomes too much trouble. By that point, it's dehydrated or ill or injured. Then they simply dump it somewhere, often to die. If the animal is lucky, it ends up at a wildlife center like ours. Even so, they need to know when to intervene and when to leave nature alone. I wanted to make sure the judge hearing the case was aware of these points.

When the day came, I made certain to arrive at the courthouse on time. The testimony proved quite entertaining. "I thought it would be pretty," the woman explained to the court, referring to the earrings. "You can get a little kid's ears pierced. What's the difference between a person's ears and a baby deer's?" When a reporter from the James Madison University student newspaper took a picture of one of the defendants, she responded with an obscene gesture—a photo the newspaper was only too happy to publish on its front page.

Ultimately, the cruelty charge was dropped when the women agreed to the illegal-possession-of-wildlife charge. They were fined the exact amount of money I calculated it cost us to house and treat Earring Boy until his release, which was then paid to the WCV in reimbursement. I'd been looking forward to offering my testimony, and when they cut the deal, I felt more than a little disappointed. The two women remained incredulous about the charges to the end.

Earring Boy thrived. Early that fall, when he weighed about sixty pounds and had lost his baby spots, he was released in a remote wooded part of Augusta County not far from the West Virginia line, along with six other juvenile deer that we'd raised as a group. They bounded off into the piney woods together, white tails held high, a signal to each other but also a good-bye to us. The group would stay together for a while, to help each other watch for predators—

and for women bearing earrings. But eventually, they would disperse and mature into adult deer.

Watching the fawns disappear into the woods, I felt a mix of emotions. Veterinarians can't help but become attached to the animals they work with, be they companion animals like cats and dogs or zoo animals like lions and tigers. But wildlife rehabilitation work is a special field. The goal of veterinarians who choose to work in this setting is to release their patients back into the wild, never to see them again. These patients rarely say thank you. More often than not, they prefer to strike out with tooth, hoof, and talon in an effort to escape—without a backward glance.

Wildlife rehabilitation veterinarians don't get many kisses from puppies. But that white tail held high, when a successfully rehabilitated deer bounds off into the woods on its way back to a life in the wild, is a pretty sweet reward in itself.

ABOUT THE AUTHOR

Ned Gentz received his doctor of veterinary medicine degree from Colorado State University in 1990 and completed an internship in zoo, wildlife, and exotic animal medicine at Kansas State University. Since 2000, he has been associate veterinarian and research coordinator at the Albuquerque Biological Park in Albuquerque, New Mexico. Previously he was director of veterinary services at the Wildlife Center of Virginia, where Animal Planet routinely filmed him at work for the television series *Wildlife Emergency*. He also served as a clinical instructor of zoo and wildlife medicine at Cornell University. Dr. Gentz is board certified by the American College of Zoological Medicine. In his current position, he volunteers his time as the consulting veterinarian for the Zuni tribe's Eagle Rescue Program. He finds this work especially inspiring.

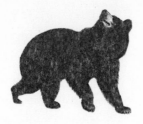

Kachina's Bones

by Becky Yates, MS, DVM

Martine called me late on a Friday afternoon from her vacation house in Arizona.

"Becky, my dear, I need you to come right away. Something is wrong with little Kachina."

Honestly, the last thing I wanted to do was drive five hours from California to Arizona to see a bear cub. I clicked my cell phone off and asked myself for the hundredth time, "Why do I work for this place, and why is it always on a weekend?" Plus, we already had more than enough animals.

Twenty years earlier, in 1976, Martine bought a piece of land north of Los Angeles, inside the boundaries of the Angeles National Forest, and established the Wildlife Waystation, a home for illegal or discarded pets. She took in leopards, jaguars, African lions, mountain lions, bobcats, bears,

coyotes, llamas, deer, hawks—even tortoises. When a research facility closed down on the East Coast, she built caging
for dozens of homeless chimps. She made room for a pride of
ligers (lion-tiger crosses) someone had bred in Idaho. Every
spring, our hospital ward filled up with baby opossums.

The call about the bear cub frustrated me. The motto at
the bottom of the Waystation entrance sign read "No Animal
Turned Away." That was an understatement. We needed
more equipment and supplies for the clinic, to say nothing of
more staff. I missed my weekends. A day off once in a while
would also be cool.

It wasn't a wild cub, I learned, but a cub from the pet in-
dustry. Someone in Arizona was breeding black bears to sell
as pets. I knew Martine well enough to know I had no choice
but to go. She wasn't asking me to make the trip; she was
telling me. On paper, I was her licensed veterinarian, even
though I'd started teaching part-time. We were trying to find
someone who could take over the bulk of my clinical duties,
especially these emergency calls.

That Friday, still annoyed, I alerted Silvio, the other
Waystation vet, and we grabbed our equipment and headed
out across the desert toward Arizona. He drove as I searched
for a radio station. I settled on country music, the only clear
signal I could find. Silvio later told me this style of music was
new to his ears; he's called it "desert music" ever since.

Why did I stay at the Waystation? I wondered again as we
cruised along. Of course, the animals were the main reason. I
knew them all, their names and their medical histories.
I regularly walked the Waystation grounds just to visit my
patients, old and new. The mostly Mexican staff was a

good group. They could rise to almost any occasion. I'd also grown attached to the place itself: simple chain-link enclosures clustered on the floor of a beautiful canyon. Martine tells a great story about how she first heard of the property from a drunk in a bar and rode up the canyon on horseback to see it.

Martine was another reason I'd stayed at the Waystation. Not only did she know her stuff, she could charm just about anyone into working his or her butt off for homeless animals. People who'd never imagined cleaning up after an animal found themselves mucking out cages, thanks to Martine. She'd never told me much about her background, only that her dad had been a diplomat and they'd traveled a lot to Africa when she was little. That must have been how she fell in love with the animal world.

Late that evening, I stood looking at a tiny black bear cub in Martine's backyard. The bear couldn't walk. When Martine picked it up, it barely responded. We guessed it was two months old and about ten pounds. The cub's stumpy little front legs were drawn in close to her chest and she whimpered whenever she moved. With each breath, her face wrinkled. She could barely keep her eyes open, and what I could see of them looked dull and listless.

Martine sat down with the cub in her lap so I could examine it. Tough as she could be, she always softened when she had an animal in her arms. She cooed at the bear but it seemed to ignore her. She insisted it had been fine during the past week, ever since a local man, hearing that Martine ran a wildlife rehabilitation facility, had dropped it off at her house. She'd named the little female Kachina, after the Hopi

Indian woodcarvings, and planned to bring her to LA when Kachina got a bit bigger.

I asked Martine for Kachina's history again. The cub had been cranky that morning, not drinking her milk, and then stopped putting any weight on her right front leg. That's when Martine had called me. Now Kachina was unable to use her left front leg.

At first, I suspected the cub had a fever. The problem could be a quick onset of some kind of bacterial or viral infection or an infectious disease affecting the joints or brain. But Kachina's temperature was normal. Palpating her front legs, I could feel they were thick and swollen. We needed an X-ray, though at that hour I had no clue where to get one. Luckily, Martine knew everyone in town. Within an hour, Silvio, Kachina, and I were being escorted into the back room of a small animal vet clinic.

The owner of the clinic seemed a bit alarmed—maybe he hadn't heard me say over the phone that the patient was a bear cub. Soon we had an anesthetic mask over Kachina's face, and after a few breaths, the isoflurane gas worked perfectly. This was the easy part. We snapped a few films and had our answer: both of the cub's front legs—the bones above her elbows—were broken.

My thoughts gelled quickly. A young animal, acutely non–weight bearing on the right and left front legs, with bilateral humeral fractures...I looked again at the radiographs. Not only were the bones fractured, they were abnormal. The outer walls give bones their strength; they should appear thick and robust on an X-ray. In Kachina's X-rays, virtually every bone in her body appeared paper-thin.

Her tiny skeleton didn't have the strength to support her weight and had fractured under the stress. Why? There must be something missing from her diet, I thought. This bear must have been getting the wrong kind of food.

I called Martine on her cell phone—she'd gone out somewhere. She was worried about Kachina but wasn't the sort of person who stood around waiting for answers. Anyway, I had Silvio with me, and she knew I'd call her with a full report.

"Martine, what kind of milk are you giving this bear?" I asked, trying not to sound accusatory. Baby carnivores require a specific type of milk. Martine knew this, of course, as she had raised dozens of young carnivores over the past several decades and was good at it.

"The same formula that came with her. She'd been taking it very well until late yesterday, as I told you before. It's in a plastic container back at the house. Why, what did you find?" The pitch of her voice rose a notch. She'd already become attached to this cub.

"Both her front legs are broken, the bones above the elbow." While I spoke to Martine, Silvio began gathering bandage material.

"Well, that would explain why she's cranky and doesn't want to eat," Martine answered calmly, her emotions back in check. "What do we do to fix this?"

Her optimistic tone didn't fit the situation—in my mind, anyway. It wasn't as if we just needed to suture a wound closed. I answered quickly, "We're going to have to put a cast on both legs, maybe even on her entire upper body. She's still anesthetized. I have to go."

Silvio and I agreed that the only option for stabilizing the thin bones was a cast. It would have to be enormous in spite of the cub's small size. After years in practice, this would be the first time we'd had to put a whole torso cast on any animal other than a lizard (but that's another story). When we finished, Kachina looked pitiful. The entire upper half of her body was encased in white casting material, with her tiny furry rear end and legs sticking out the back and her head sticking out the top. We tried to put a slight bend in the cast so her front legs were not totally straight. Our biggest worry was whether she could breathe normally, since the cast undoubtedly put some pressure on her chest. We decided the best thing we could do for the cub was to keep her calm.

As soon as Kachina woke up, we mixed some Valium in honey. No bear refuses honey. She took it readily. Two hours later, back at Martine's house, she took her bottle. A good sign. The plan at that point was to have Martine keep Kachina quiet in the cast while her bones healed. The next morning, Silvio and I headed back to LA with some blood samples.

Halfway home, I realized I hadn't looked at the milk powder label. I called Martine and asked her to check it. "Becky, as I told you, it says Commercial Bear Milk Powder. It came with the bear."

"Does it say anything on the label?" I asked.

"Becky, it says Commercial Bear Milk Powder," Martine repeated, sounding irritated.

—

A week later, I drove back to check on Kachina and to get a sample of the milk powder. We'd run the cub's blood samples and found an abnormal inverted ratio of calcium to phosphorous. These results confirmed the diagnosis: Kachina's bones were thin from a condition called metabolic bone disease. While young carnivores need to consume both calcium and phosphorous, there is normally more calcium than phosphorous in their mothers' milk. When they start eating the flesh of other animals, they get these minerals from bones and cartilage as well as from meat. If they don't get the right proportions of minerals, their bones cannot mineralize normally. This is a classic disease that occurs in captivity when the wrong type of milk or meat without bones is fed to a carnivore. It can happen in lions, tigers—and bears.

Walking into the backyard, I expected to find a sedated and immobile bear. Instead, Kachina was a ball of energy. She'd figured out how to walk by using her cast like a sled. Propelling herself with her back legs, she took corners by tipping her cast to angle around the turns. To my surprise and great relief, Kachina had adapted beautifully to her confinement. This was an endearing animal. Encouraged by her energy, we changed her diet: no more mystery milk powder. We gave the cub a small amount of a commercial zoo diet made for bears called "omnivore chow," a fancy type of dog kibble. She seemed to like it. Our plan was to wean her off milk with the hope that solid food—and the correct amounts of calcium and phosphorous—would help her bones catch up with the rest of her body.

I no longer minded the house calls to another state. We were definitely making progress, and Kachina was no longer in pain. On my third trip, four weeks after we'd put her in the body cast, I noticed the bandage material was starting to break down, and also that she was growing out of it. The better the cub felt, the more stress she put on the cast; it wouldn't last much longer. But before we replaced it, we wanted to see how the bones were healing. We arranged to go back to the local vet clinic and take another set of radiographs. This time we simply laid Kachina on the table and took pictures of her front legs through the cast.

Expecting to see progress, we were stunned by the results. The bones were not healing at all. We could barely even see them. They were disappearing. Maybe our cast was too good, so supportive that it had removed all the stress on her bones, something they needed in order to mineralize.

I had a sinking feeling this bear wouldn't make it—that the bones would never heal. Though Kachina seemed to feel fine, it was only the cast that was holding her little body together. We decided to go ahead and change the cast, which meant anesthetizing her after all. Luckily, bears are pretty easy anesthetic patients, and she slept quietly while we took new pictures and replaced the cast. No one said much. It didn't seem right to put this great wad of material around the cub's small body if it wasn't going to help cure her. I left for LA with very little hope.

We had lots of discussion at that point. Silvio and I reviewed the X-rays and the blood work results again, and set up a meeting with Martine. She wanted us to take the cub to an orthopedist. "Spare no expense" seemed to be the Waystation's unwritten motto, even though funds were always tight. We explained that the bones weren't strong enough to support surgical repair using plates or pins. Martine wouldn't accept this answer. So we took more

X-rays using a special technique, digital radiography, in order to improve the image quality. We sent them to a specialist. The answer was what Silvio and I had expected: no surgical options.

We pored through books, made phone calls, talked to several other vets, and tried to get the results of the milk analysis. Though they still weren't available, we had to believe that the original formula had been inappropriate nutrition for the bear's healthy growth. Kachina's diet was now as balanced as we could make it.

But maybe it was too balanced? Maybe we should try providing an imbalance in the other direction—giving her more calcium than she needed. This approach carried some risk because excess calcium can build up in the kidneys, but we felt it was worth a try. The medicine of choice is called Neocalglucon, a calcium-rich, sweet syrup made for children who don't like milk. We give it to birds when they're having trouble laying eggs. Kachina loved it.

Two weeks later, I made yet another house call to Arizona. We repeated the visit to the local vet clinic. By now, everyone knew Kachina and her traveling vets. She'd become a favorite with all who'd met her. With the cast off, I carefully palpated the fracture sites. They were still mobile. It was as if we'd made no progress. The word "euthanasia" loomed in my mind. I put on a new cast, but decided that it was time to have a difficult conversation with Martine. It wasn't fair to put the little bear through all of this for much longer if we couldn't heal her.

Back at the house, Martine poured a glass of wine for herself and handed me a beer. "Becky," she began in her familiar,

demanding tone, "why would you even think about euthaniz-
ing Kachina when she is running all over the yard like a happy
three-year-old? The animal looks fine. Can't we just give her
time?"

Basically, Martine was telling me that putting the cub
down was not an option. It wasn't what I wanted to do anyway, so I didn't react to her tone. I sipped my beer silently.
I remembered the advice of an orthopedic surgeon in
vet school: if you have a cat or a small dog with a broken
leg, just put it in a box. It will heal. The orthopedist meant:
confine the animal to minimize its activity. Surgery isn't
the answer. Also radiographic changes lag behind actual
changes in the bone. The callus around a fracture site can be
fairly complete but it doesn't mineralize completely for
weeks.

Silvio and I talked about the cub again. Kachina's appetite
had been great, she was growing, and we saw no sign that the
bear was in pain. We all agreed to give her a few more weeks.

Something was different about the cub on my next visit.
She seemed stronger, bigger, and brighter. She needed yet another cast. Once again, we took radiographs, not expecting
to see anything positive. But finally, there they were—the
outlines of her bones!

Kachina was lucky that it was Martine who had taken
charge of her recovery. She'd insisted that we give the bear
more time, and she was right. I learned a lesson from
Martine that day, one I realized I'd also been taught many
years ago in vet school: remember to look at your patient,
not the test results.

In this business, so many animals don't make it through

rehabilitation that when there's a good outcome, you're pleasantly surprised—in this case overjoyed. I truly hadn't thought this little bear would live. When I called the company that made the so-called bear milk, I talked to them until they hung up on me. They weren't about to take responsibility, even though analysis proved their product was completely wrong for a bear.

After working at the Waystation on and off for fifteen years, I recently left that job in order to teach full-time. But I visit when I can. Katrina is up to two hundred pounds and lives with another female bear. The image of that little cub in a whole-body cast sliding around Martine's backyard still makes me smile. Thanks to her, and the Waystation, this bear has a good home.

ABOUT THE AUTHOR

Rebecca A. Yates spent her early years tending to small creatures like birds, lizards, tortoises, and insects in Los Angeles. She received her bachelor's degree at Humboldt State University, her master of science at California State University, Dominguez Hills, and her degree in veterinary medicine at University of California, Davis. After finishing vet school, Dr. Yates briefly cared for cats and dogs until discovering her true passion in zoo animal and wildlife medicine. She spent nearly ten years working with a variety of wild animal species—including native wildlife—at the Wildlife Waystation near Los Angeles, California. She moved to the East Coast to work as staff veterinarian for two years at the National Zoo in Washington, DC, and then returned to California, resuming part-time work for the Waystation while she pursued a career in teaching. She currently teaches full-time for the veterinary technology program at Pierce College. Dr. Yates can often be seen riding her off-road unicycle up steep canyon roads.

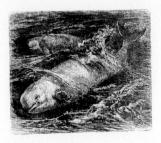

Raising Kayavak

by Jeff Boehm, DVM

At the time (2000), no one in the world had successfully raised a five-month-old orphaned baby beluga whale. Our choices were decidedly few. We could create an artificial whale milk formula for the calf, attempt to foster her onto an adult female whale who'd recently lost a calf, or force her through a "cold turkey" approach to weaning considerably earlier than we thought advisable. I tried to think of a fourth or fifth option as I hurried from O'Hare Airport to Shedd Aquarium on Chicago's lakefront. I wished I'd never left for California. Then again, I'd been looking forward to visiting family for the holidays.

The whale trainers and the on-duty veterinarian, Dr. Annelisa Kilbourn, first noticed something wrong the day before, late on Christmas morning. The calf's mother,

Immiayuk, was acting a bit strange. Observations intensified and concern mounted as the day wore on. Immi appeared lethargic and uninterested in her training sessions. Annelisa called me and we agreed that I should race back. The aquarium staff quickly moved into high gear, shifting mom and calf into a separate pool so they could keep an even closer eye on the pair. Next, they began the slow process of lowering the pool water. The plan was to examine Immi this morning while I flew halfway across the country.

As I sat on the plane, possible causes for Immi's changes played out in my mind over and over, from a simple behavioral problem to acute infection. Anxious to get back, I tried to distract myself by studying the other passengers. I wondered if any of my fellow travelers had started the day as I had, with no travel plans whatsoever. It was a safe bet no one else was answering an emergency call about a sick whale and her five-month-old baby.

The moment we landed, I called for an update. The tearful voice on the other end of the phone confirmed my worst fear: Immi had died. My heart went out to the animal care staff. I imagined their faces, strained with concern and grief. Everyone would be discussing what needed to be done next. The baby whale would soon be very hungry. We had some difficult, critical decisions to make—and fast.

By the time I got to the aquarium, night had fallen and the clock was ticking for little Kayavak. Annelisa and I met with the curators to talk about what to do next. The calf could dehydrate and weaken quickly without a source of milk. At the same time, we needed to determine the probable cause for her mother's death. It could have been an isolated event, or it could be something that threatened the health of the other whales, including this precious calf. The difficult task of performing a postmortem examination on Immi—a 1,700-pound animal—would require our complete attention for several hours, and we'd need most of the crew helping. But the 250-pound baby also needed us, and that meant getting close to her. Not a routine proposition.

We elected to drop the water level in the baby's pool right away, so that we could perform a physical exam and give her fluids. Administering an electrolyte solution to her orally would at least reduce the risk of dehydration while we sorted out our options. As soon as the water level dropped to a few feet, staff climbed down into the pool and slowly gathered around Kayavak. She proved to be a compliant patient, allowing trainers to gently restrain her in their arms as they knelt in the water. I passed a flexible tube into Kayavak's mouth and then her stomach while Annelisa poured the fluids in, using a funnel.

When we finished, the little whale swam away slowly. She'd been through a tremendous amount over the past twenty-four hours, and it seemed as if she would accept whatever we chose to do for her. We made tentative plans to repeat the calf's fluid treatments every three or four hours over the next day to maintain her hydration. This would give us time to assess why Immi had died and formulate a plan for Kayavak's nutrition.

One of our options—seemingly the most straightforward—was to jump into the business of making baby whale milk. Every mammal requires its own milk formula. These don't come standardized, and figuring out what works best requires some trial and error. We certainly could not use human, dog, or horse milk formula for a whale calf. Like all marine mammals, these little guys have a huge demand for calorie-dense, fat-rich milk. We might be able to use commercially available milk powders as a base, but we'd need to buy massive amounts and then figure out just the right mix. Or we could use what others had used to raise orphaned dolphins: heavy whipping cream blended with herring fillets.

We got on the phone to search for more information and determine exactly what we'd need to pull this off. If we chose to pursue this course and raise the calf on formula, it would be a first for a beluga whale. The trick would be to formulate a whale milk "recipe" that would get the biggest caloric bang for our liquid buck. Rather than the ounces per day required by a human infant, we'd be dealing with whale-sized gallons per day! And she would need more all the time as she grew. I wondered if our industrial-strength blender was ready to go.

Getting the milk into Kayavak posed even greater concerns. Even if we could teach this baby how to nurse from a bottle, we couldn't do it soon enough to get the calories she needed today, or even within several days. So we would have to start by placing the tube down her throat into her stomach and pouring the milk through a funnel, the same method we'd used for the electrolyte fluids. Annelisa and I didn't need to be involved—the technicians and trainers could do this step. But how often?

The calf had been nursing from her mother every twenty minutes to one hour, and we couldn't come close to matching that frequency with stomach tubing. Realistically, we could tube-feed her three times a day. We also didn't know exactly how much she drank each time she nursed, though we guessed it must have been several ounces. This meant large volumes of milk—up to a gallon—would have to be delivered at each of the three feedings.

We knew we could succeed with this method at the beginning. Kayavak had tolerated the earlier fluids just fine. But would the calf continue to cooperate, or would she begin to resist us? Would the stress of being handled create new problems? Pneumonia loomed as a possible complication of stomach tubing because we'd be putting such a large volume into her stomach each time. Whales breathe through a physically separate and protected blowhole. Even so, if we overfilled her stomach or she struggled during the tube-feeding process, we could inadvertently get milk flowing back up and around the airway into the wrong place—her lungs. As in any animal, that would be a serious and potentially fatal problem.

We would eventually teach her to drink from a bottle and stop the stomach tubing. But how many days or even weeks would that take?

Meanwhile, our veterinary pathology team had begun the postmortem exam on Immi. Annelisa and I stopped in to check on their progress frequently. To our frustration, the exam revealed no clear answers. When an animal dies unexpectedly, as Immi did, we hope to at least learn why. There are few things more frustrating than not being able to determine the cause of death. Sometimes a preliminary examination leads to a sudden "Aha!" moment in which an obvious answer is found, but that wasn't the case here. As the pathologists continued their work, moving from a gross examination on to the process of evaluating tissues microscopically, we had no definitive explanation for what happened. And we had very few clues.

We agreed that the most likely explanation for a fatal illness that occurred so quickly was an overwhelming bacterial infection. If we were right about this diagnosis in the mother, what did we need to consider about the calf? We hedged our bets and added antibiotics to the emerging treatment regimen for Kayavak. As to the source of the infection, we began a series of tests to look for unusual bacteria in the food or water. It would take at least twenty-four hours before we'd have any results. Eventually, we confirmed that Immi died from erysipelas, an overwhelming bacterial infection known to cause rapid death in marine mammals.

Immi's loss hit us all hard. She had been one of the aquarium's first beluga whales; Kayavak was her first calf. This pair of charismatic, intelligent, and highly social animals had also become Chicago's media darlings. The staff and public adored them. Together they represented the success of our beluga breeding program. Now one was gone forever and the other was in trouble. We also worried about the rest of the aquarium's beluga collection. We could only hope that what had killed Immi would not strike again.

We took frequent breaks from Kayavak to look in on the rest of the whales. We also wondered what they sensed or understood about the events of the last few days. Experts who study elephants have observed a mourning process when a herd member dies. Was this occurring with our whales? Does a whale grieve as we do? We didn't know. But we did know one thing: we wouldn't let them out of our sight. We needed to reassure ourselves that everyone was healthy.

Our second option for Kayavak was to foster her onto another whale, Puiji. As the night wore on, we paid particular attention to this female who had given birth a few weeks before Immi. Sadly, her calf survived for only a short time. We couldn't be certain, but Puiji would very likely resume lactating if presented with a calf.

This option appealed to us for several reasons. Not only would the calf be drinking the real thing, she would have the companionship during her infancy of a mother whale. It's not surprising to see a beluga calf nursing well into its second year. Though Kayavak had hit every milestone, at five months old her natural weaning time was still many, many months away.

But here too there were challenges to consider. Kayavak had never actually been in the same habitat with Puiji. The two might not bond. The adult whale could be aggressive or uninterested. She might not produce any milk. How much time could we give these two to forge a relationship before we'd feel compelled to intervene and feed Kayavak? And could we determine if the calf's nutritional needs were being met, when and if nursing began? Ultimately, this option left a lot to chance. We had to decide how comfortable we were with the idea of letting go. The calf's fate would be largely out of our control in this scenario.

Another pool drop just after midnight to give the calf a second dose of fluids left staff tired. Kayavak, on the other hand, acted as if the night had just begun. She looked for attention and repeatedly swam over to the trainers stationed poolside. Clearly, she wanted them in the water with her.

We took her cue and started a new rotation: swimming with Kayavak. Trainers lined up for this assignment. It hardly felt like work. They swam alongside the curious whale or floated on rafts within reach, allowing her to brush their hands as she passed nearby. If Kayavak was grieving, she was also pragmatic. She learned very quickly where she could get the attention she wanted. These wet-suited people might not be great swimmers, but they were acceptable as new companions.

I often marvel at how much we know about these animals, yet how much more we need to learn. Although you won't find the definitive textbook on rearing orphaned beluga calves on your library shelf, you will find, among the ranks of veterinarians the world over, a willingness to innovate, to extrapolate, and to share experiences. We tapped into the aquarium world network again to explore our third option for Kayavak: weaning her straight onto fish.

No one had tried this approach in a whale calf. But we heard several encouraging stories about dolphins. Young dolphins will start eating whole fish even while continuing to nurse. We heard about one dolphin successfully weaned from nursing at six months of age. Although the information trickling in from our colleagues did not exactly amount to a peer-reviewed scientific paper, it did represent the most intriguing and, in many ways, the least risky of our three choices. Conventional wisdom was that a six-month-old whale needs milk. But if a six-month-old dolphin could survive on fish, why couldn't a whale calf? Plus, we were sure we could train Kayavak to eat.

We met to share our ideas. Veterinarians, curators, and trainers pooled their thoughts and expertise while the aquarium's director looked on. We called more experts, combed the literature, and borrowed a page or two from domestic animal medicine. There was no clear right answer. The only wrong answer was inaction, and so we moved quickly.

By the first light of morning, we had our decision. We would abruptly wean Kayavak onto solid food. With this approach, we'd have control over her nutrition and intake; we could weigh her routinely, monitor her for illness, and still have the option of providing fluids and milk by tube-feeding if necessary. We'd blend aggressive veterinary medicine, expert animal care, and intensive animal training. We'd teach Kayavak how to eat and then wean her from us—sooner rather than later.

Kayavak ate her first fish on December 27. At that session, she received three herring. Though she gave us a quizzical look, she seemed no worse for the experience. By day's end, she'd received two and a half kilograms of fish, or about 20 percent of what we'd calculated she would need each day. We continued to supplement her with fluids and treat her with antibiotics. The next day she was up to three and a half kilos. By week's end, she was approaching trainers for food as well as attention. After three weeks, she was eagerly taking fish from the trainers.

As expected, the whale lost weight at first, but she remained bright-eyed, energetic, and responsive to her human caretakers. She handled her new diet well, and her appetite was growing. After two months, the calf had surpassed her original weight. She was ready to meet the other whales.

Before Immi's death, Kayavak and her mother had lived together in a pool separate from the other belugas. They had access to each other only across netted gates. We wanted to minimize the chance of complications during birth and limit the risk of aggression toward the newborn. Mother belugas tend to be very protective of their babies. Additionally, female whales will sometimes try to steal another mother's calf. Now we followed a step-by-step plan to introduce Kayavak slowly to the adults, one at a time, over a period of months. Each time we opened the gate that connected her pool to the adult pool and began an introduction to a new whale, we felt considerable trepidation.

Immi had been the dominant animal in the pod before the birth of this calf. Whale social behavior depends largely on hierarchy; we wondered if Kayavak would benefit from her mother's prior status. Such social dynamics are complicated, however, and what we understood about the rankings of our beluga community was likely just the tip of the iceberg. With Immi gone, things could have shifted in ways that would be hard to predict.

Sure enough, despite the role her mother once played, Kayavak wasn't accorded any special status. On the contrary, she entered the pod at the bottom of the pecking order, and there were times when the older whales showed aggression toward her. But, ultimately, she held her own. Gradually she learned to navigate the society of her new pod and became a solid part of the community.

Even so, Kayavak maintained a bond with all of us. She

would throw a glance toward her human companions now and then, as if to let us know she'd made it. We felt as though she were looking back at us with a wink and a nod. Our relationship with her continues to be a special one. Now a young adult, Kayavak is an integral part of the beluga group at the aquarium. A guest wouldn't be able to pick her out from among the other animals, but every member of the aquarium staff can identify her at a glance.

Kayavak's case, with its sad and startling beginning but successful resolution, made a lasting impression on me. Of all the lessons we learned that winter—about nutrition and infectious disease, behavior and environmental enrichment, tough decision making, and acceptance of risk—perhaps the most powerful were the ones we learned from Kayavak. She taught us about adaptability and survival. This endearing whale sought the care and companionship she needed to survive, and we happily provided it.

ABOUT THE AUTHOR

Jeff Boehm is a graduate of the University of California, San Diego, where he received his bachelor's degree, and the University of California, Davis, where he received his degree in veterinary medicine. He completed an internship in small animal medicine in Southern California and then worked as a veterinary clinician at the Los Angeles Zoo. Since 1992, Dr. Boehm has worked at the John G. Shedd Aquarium in Chicago, where he is currently the senior vice president for animal health and conservation science and the Louis Family Conservation chair. In this position, he oversees the aquarium's veterinary division, a variety of conservation science initiatives, and a Great Lakes conservation program. Dr. Boehm has a keen interest in aquatic conservation, specifically the role that zoos and aquariums play in fieldwork and research, and ultimately in public awareness.

II

Technology Helps

MRI scans produce excellent images in turtles, lasers limit blood loss during surgery in fish, ultrasound studies can detect heart disease in gorillas, orthopedic surgery works well in birds, and root canals are readily performed on lions, tigers, and bears. All of these animals are monitored during anesthesia with pulse oximetry, a measure of heart rate and blood oxygen saturation. With the help of medical technology, zoo vets arrive at diagnoses earlier, predict outcomes more accurately, and treat symptoms more successfully.

Given the range of species and potential problems in zoological medicine, there's sometimes a first-time technological solution. It might be the application of familiar technology to an unfamiliar species, or the replacement of a traditional medical tool with a newer one.

The process of applying such techniques in wild animals, however, is anything but routine. Even the simplest technique may require a degree of modification, depending on the species. In order to make such adjustments, we collaborate with experts in other medical fields, including domestic and large animal veterinarians, physicians, medical technicians, and veterinary and human dentists. Adding to the challenge, most of our patients must be restrained, anesthetized, or trained for months before they will tolerate even simple technology-based procedures. A sick octopus in need of a set of X-rays, for example, requires three sets of hands and a barrel of water, with a water-soluble anesthetic available as backup.

Radiography, the production of images using X-rays, is a good example of the application of medical technology in zoological medicine. In both humans and animals, bones and other cartilaginous structures appear white, internal organs appear various shades of gray, and air-filled structures appear black. X-ray images readily show the patient's skeleton, including its teeth, and the outline of major structures such as the heart, lungs, intestinal tract, liver, kidneys, and bladder.

The size and density of the animal determines the type of cassette that holds the film and the power required to produce the image. Dental film, the kind we humans bite down on while sitting in a dentist's chair, works fine for whole-body images of tiny animals like hummingbirds, small fish, and frogs. We use standard-sized X-ray cassettes for small mammals like meerkats and monkeys, or for various body parts of larger animals—the thorax of a wolf, the abdomen of a tiger, the skull of a tapir, or the hoof of a zebra. Whether the exam is performed in a fully equipped veterinary hospital or in the field, the patient is almost always anesthetized or lightly restrained.

Interpreting the X-ray images poses another challenge. Experience and knowledge of comparative radiographic anatomy are crucial to accurate interpretation, and even then opinions may vary. The radiographic anatomy of a gorilla most resembles that of a human, but with quite a few differences, not the least of which is the size of the hands and skull relative to the body and the presence of air-filled sacs located beneath the neck and in each armpit. Birds have air sacs too, and some of their bones are full of air cavities. But there are many differences among these species as well. An X-ray of a parrot looks very different from that of a hawk.

With the arrival of digital photography and digital radiography, many zoo vets use e-mail to send radiographs to experts at other institutions for another opinion. As a whole, our profession has been quick to take advantage of the Internet. Not only do we use this tool for communication, it's often the first place we look for the latest medical technology.

Zoo vets show their low- and high-tech creativity in the next group of stories: horseshoes give a rhino relief, fiber-optic instruments help pandas, massive portable life-support systems transport whale sharks halfway around the world, orthopedic surgery helps a falcon, and frogs benefit from a new anesthetic method.

Lucy H. Spelman, DVM

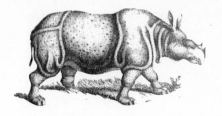

The Rhino with Glue-On Shoes

by Lucy H. Spelman, DVM

There had to be a better way to deal with this rhino's feet. Blood dripped from Mohan's foot pads as veterinarians and technicians worked furiously to carve away diseased tissue. These were not small feet—each one measured about ten inches in diameter. A growing pile of soiled gauze and towels littered the floor. Next, bandages would go on. Then we'd roll the rhino over to work on the other side. The blood didn't worry us. Even if Mo lost a few pints during the trim, the 5,000-pound animal wouldn't know it.

In an odd sort of way, we were glad to see red. The blackened, unhealthy tissue wedged between his toes and into the cracks of his soles had outgrown its vascular supply. His back feet were the worst. We trimmed off the outside layers until we got down to healthy tissue, which bled profusely. I watched the foot-trimming team for a minute or so, long enough to gauge how much more anesthesia time they needed. Then I turned my attention back to the rhino. Though we'd done this procedure many times before, it still felt like a big deal to put him under anesthesia.

At thirty-two, Mo was one of the oldest greater one-horned rhinos in captivity and genetically valuable. When he arrived at the National Zoo, in Washington, DC, in 1998, three years before, everyone hoped that he and Mechi, our female, would breed. He had never bred, and we knew he had a history of foot problems. Unfortunately, the pattern continued. Though the two seemed compatible, Mechi showed more interest in Mo than he did in her and his feet continued to deteriorate.

Fortunately, Mo handled anesthesia well. He'd stand still for the darting and slump to the ground ten minutes later when the drug took effect. Sometimes he'd go down in the middle of the enclosure, which made it easy. Other times he'd jam his great nose in a corner. We'd reposition him using a few ropes and about a dozen people. I'd put a catheter in his ear, start him on an IV filled with muscle relaxant, and then put a rubber hose up one nostril to deliver oxygen. The minute we had our first set of vital signs, the rest of the team got to work and the trimming began.

Given his age and the ever-present risk of complications, I tended to keep Mo's anesthesia on the light side. At the slightest indication of a problem, I could quickly reverse him (wake him up). Since this strategy meant that a loud noise or bright light could cause him to stir, we covered his eyes with a cloth drape, packed his ears with gauze, and kept a syringe full of anesthetic at the ready.

I lifted the rhino's blindfold and peered into his big dark

eyes. Even anesthetized animals have some sort of facial expression that offers a clue to their mental state. Mo stared past me, unblinking. His eyelids were stretched wide open, a side effect of the anesthetic, just as they should be at this stage in the procedure. I applied a bit more "eye goop," a sterile ophthalmic ointment, to protect the surface of his corneas, and replaced the cover.

Checking for an ear twitch, I tickled the hairs in his upside ear. No reaction. Good. A chunk of brown wax stuck to my gloved finger. I fiddled with the hose delivering oxygen. No snort or change in breathing. Our monitors showed a steady heart rate and good blood oxygen saturation. I slipped my hands into his mouth to check his jaw tone; the muscles resisted. He'd definitely need a supplement of anesthetic before the team rolled him onto his other side. Otherwise, he might be able to kick out, or even try to get up. I also got a whiff of bad breath. Maybe we could float (file) his teeth if we had time.

"How's it going, Paul?" I asked. A large animal veterinarian, Dr. Paul Anikis had long since become a vital member of our zoo's consulting team. He'd driven ninety miles into the city from the Virginia countryside early this morning. It was now just past seven-thirty AM.

"These feet are a mess, Lucy, they really are. We're gonna try perfusing him today, the way we do in horses. The back feet, anyway. I don't think oral antibiotics will even touch this stuff." Paul shook his head. "It seems like these toe pads are the problem. They've got to be really sore. If we can get a cephalosporin IV in there, it'll reduce all that swelling. We're mixing some up now."

When Mo's feet needed trimming, the rhino's entire

demeanor changed. Normally, he never missed a chance for a food treat or a belly scratch. Erin, one of his keepers, had trained him to stand next to the bars of his indoor enclosure, close enough that she could reach in and work on his feet. While the other keepers distracted him with bits of sweet potato, Erin could give him a mini-pedicure.

But she could only trim bits of the overgrown tissue. Rhinos have three hooved toes on each foot. The skin between Mo's toes and the soles of his feet grew abnormally. At a certain point, this tissue fissured and cracked, allowing dirt and bacteria in and causing infection. Then it swelled. Mo couldn't stand without pinching this infected skin. It hurt. Because the problem affected all four feet, we didn't always see lameness, but his overall behavior changed. He avoided standing for long periods of time. Instead of enjoying his shower for an hour, for example, he would lie down in the middle of his enclosure. His eyelids and ears drooped. He would rarely come over to the bars. At that point, we'd schedule him for a complete trim under anesthesia.

I knelt back down next to the rhino's huge head, and watched again as Paul worked on the feet. He used a rope to fashion a tourniquet just below the rhino's tarsal-metatarsal (ankle) joint. Using a short piece of tubing with a needle on the end, a butterfly catheter, he quickly found a vein and injected the medicine. It would flood the tissue of the foot and stay there until he removed the rope. He followed that with some lidocaine, a local anesthetic, to ensure that Mo wouldn't feel anything.

For the bandage, Paul started with a combination of cotton and gauze wrap, covered by stretchy material called

Vetwrap. We'd been through a fair amount of trial and error with this last step. Our first set of bandages stayed on for only a few hours. Mo got his feet wet and kicked them off. We wanted the bandages to last a day or two, long enough to keep his feet clean immediately after the trim. The answer? Duct tape, of course: the wide gray sticky tape used to patch holes in just about anything. The brand in our kit that day had a clever brand name, Duck Tape, with a picture of a yellow duck standing in a puddle of water.

The team waited for me to give the rhino a bit more anesthetic and then pushed him up onto his sternum and over onto the other side, folding his legs under his body. Mo's heavy head rested in my lap during the shift, temporarily pinning me to the floor. Adjusting the blindfold, I checked his eyes again: no change. The extra dose had worked perfectly. I couldn't resist giving his neck a light pat. His rough skin felt like concrete with a little flex, reminding me of Rudyard Kipling's description: bumpy plates of armor.

Thirty minutes later, just as Paul finished bandaging the second rear foot, the rhino blinked and opened his eyelids extremely wide. The initial narcotic anesthetic had begun to wear off at just the right time. Minutes later, with most of the staff and equipment cleared away, I gave Mo a drug that would reverse the remaining effects of the anesthetic, took a last set of vital signs, and removed his catheter. Erin stayed with me at his head. Her shoes spattered with blood, she looked tired, having spent most of the time bent over, helping to hold Mo's feet.

"He'll feel so much better in a few days," I said quietly as we waited for the effects of the reversal drug to kick in.

"I know," Erin responded. "I just wish we didn't have to put him through this much, at his age."

As the anesthetic reversal took effect, the rhino took a huge breath and lifted his nose. We pulled out the ear gauze, removed the blindfold, and backed out of the stall. Mo heaved himself to his feet, wobbling. Watery blood dripped from his elbows. He took a few steps, shaking his bandaged feet. The duct tape held. Once again, he'd sailed through the anesthesia. When I stopped by to check him two hours later, he appeared remarkably normal.

From past experience, we knew the rhino's feet would improve after the trim. We also knew we hadn't solved anything. The infection would return within several months. In fact, Mo had been suffering from this problem for much of his life. It started long before he came to Washington, DC, while he lived at a zoo in Florida. Maybe the antibiotic perfusion would knock down the bacteria and keep them away for a bit longer this time. Like Erin, I wondered how many more times we could anesthetize him safely.

Some months later, at a veterinary conference, I attended a presentation about foot problems in rhinos, expecting to hear the familiar advice: trim and trim again; try antibiotic footbaths. Instead, the speaker, Dr. Mark Atkinson, focused on what he had learned about greater one-horned rhinos in the wild. Throughout India, Nepal, Bhutan, and Thailand, this species—also known as the Indian rhino—lives in swampy grasslands and mud wallows.

Mark recommended that zoos dramatically change the way they housed these rhinos. A pool isn't enough, he said; give these animals the swamps and mud their feet need. Take the pressure off their soles by getting them off gravel and cement floors. He also pointed out that many zoo rhinos were overweight, compounding the problem. Why weren't zoos providing the proper conditions? It was partly due to lack of understanding of what this species needs to be healthy, partly the cost of adding wallows, and partly the weather.

For nine months of the year in Washington, Mo had access to his outdoor pool and the mud around it. And he spent most of his time there. During winter, however, he lived mostly inside, protected from the cold. Mo's feet worsened within weeks of the start of wintertime housing routines.

While he spoke, Mark flashed images of normal feet from wild rhinos in Nepal alongside images of abnormal ones living in captivity. Rhinos have three toes and a main foot pad. They naturally bear most of their weight on their toenails, each analogous to a horse's hoof with a hard outer wall that extends well below a concave sole. Healthy wild rhinos are "toe walkers." Since they naturally walk on soft ground, their toenails show very little wear. Captive rhinos have short nails with flat soles that fall even with the main foot pad; they are "pad walkers."

Suddenly, Mo's real problem became crystal clear: his toenails were completely worn down from a lifetime on hard ground, exposing his soles—and then his main foot pad—to excess weight. Swampy ground might have prevented this problem, and it certainly had to be part of the long-term solution, but for now this rhino's feet were caught in a painful vicious cycle. Every time we cut the overgrown sole tissue back, it barely came even with his nails. He walked mostly on his sore soles.

I arranged for Paul to stop by to see Mo so I could show him some of the photos. He reacted to Mark's findings with a new idea.

"Okay, so let's put shoes on him," he said.

"Shoes?" I was surprised. "Paul, you're crazy. How do we do that?"

"We'll just glue 'em on. No problem. I've been putting these aluminum shoes on the US Equestrian Team dressage horses because they're light, and you don't have to put nails through their feet to keep them on. We use epoxy and a fiberglass patch. You know, the way you fix broken turtle shells. If we can just get him up off his soles and give his nails some relief, they might have a chance to grow out more normally."

"But won't we have to go back and take the shoes off at some point?" I asked, worried about the number of times we'd have to put the rhino (and ourselves) through anesthesia. The more I thought about an aluminum shoe glued onto the bottom of a rhino foot, the crazier it sounded. I imagined two scenarios: the rhino would wake up from anesthesia, tap around inside his enclosure, and throw off the shoes. Or the glue would hold them in place forever.

"Nah, he'll wear 'em off eventually. Most people probably won't even notice he has them on." Paul thought for a moment. "Send me measurements of his back feet—the really bad ones—and some tracings of his footprints, if the keepers can get them. I'll make a prefab set of shoes so the whole thing goes quickly. I think we should do this sooner rather than later, before his feet get really bad again."

We were all excited when the time came to give Mo his

new shoes. Once again, there was extensive secondary infection in his rear feet, though the front feet were not so bad. After the trimming and antibiotic perfusion, Paul pulled the shoes out of his bag. I'd visualized thick pads of some sort. Instead, they looked a lot like standard horseshoes, without the holes, and shaped a bit differently. Of course, the other difference was that Mo would wear three shoes on each back foot, one for each of his three toes.

Paul started prepping the shoes for the epoxy. He checked each one for size and shape. The shoe for the middle toes was a larger C shape than those for the smaller inner and outer toes. Since rhino toes spread out when the animal stands, the three shoes would support a fair amount of Mo's weight; his main foot pad would support the rest. The combined surface of the shoes would function as surrogate toenails.

Working at his usual rapid pace, Paul applied a thin layer of glue to the underside of each shoe. The bitter smell of adhesive filled the air. He pressed the shoe onto the sole close to the edge of the toe, and covered it with Kevlar fiberglass strips slathered in more glue. This patch acted like a Band-Aid to create a better seal and extend the life of the shoe.

Paul pressed the shoes in place for several minutes, allowing the adhesive to take hold, and then wrapped the foot lightly: no need for the heavy gray tape today. We wanted Mo to shed these bandages by nightfall so he'd be walking on his new shoes. As Paul finished side two, I said, "Hey, wow, snazzy shoes! Bet this is a first for a greater one-horned rhino."

"Yup. I'm happy with them. He should feel a lot better. Let's see how he wakes up."

Later in the morning, I came back to check on Mo. He stood drowsily eating hay. Erin smiled at him. Good old Mo—another uneventful recovery.

His bandages already off, Mo walked over to us, his feet making a light tapping sound on the concrete floor. He pushed his great one-horned nose between the bars for a piece of carrot. The eye ointment from the procedure had seeped into the skin around his eyes, making them look even rounder and darker than usual. Mo seemed exceptionally calm and relaxed, and we thought the shoes were already giving him some relief. Erin joked that he might start tap-dancing at any moment.

The shoes lasted longer than I'd imagined. Though the ones on the smaller inner and outer toes fell off by three months, the central toe shoes were still in place and doing their job for another six weeks. And although the chronic infection began its slow recurrence, Mo's nails did grow out. When he and Mechi left the zoo for a wetter, swampier exhibit and a warmer climate, we felt we'd given him a better footing for what remained of his captive-rhino life.

ABOUT THE AUTHOR

Lucy H. Spelman grew up with a menagerie of animals on an old dairy farm in rural Connecticut. While in middle school, she looked forward to "old clothes Wednesday," a day set aside by one of her teachers to explore the nature trails across the street. She earned a bachelor of arts in biology from Brown University, then her veterinary degree from the University of California, Davis, and completed her postdoctoral training at North Carolina State University. Board certified by the American College of Zoological Medicine in 1994, Dr. Spelman's work experience includes nearly ten years with the Smithsonian National Zoo, half as a clinical veterinarian and half as its director. She joined the Mountain Gorilla Veterinary Project in October 2006 as its Africa-based regional manager. Dr. Spelman enjoys sharing her work with others through all forms of media. In addition to writing, she has been filmed at work with animals in more than a dozen cable television documentaries, and has served as a consultant for various media and education divisions of Discovery Communications, Inc. "We're all in this together," she says of today's conservation challenges.

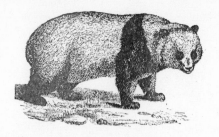

Pandas in Their Own Land

by Carlos Sanchez, DVM, MSc

In 2005, I was in Chengdu, China, preparing to perform a colonoscopy on a female giant panda with an undiagnosed intestinal disorder. This visit was the latest of several I'd made to the Chengdu Research Base of Giant Panda Breeding. My Chinese colleagues had picked out several animals with chronic illnesses, and we'd planned to give each one a complete physical under anesthesia—including endoscopy and abdominal ultrasound. This particular panda, Yaloda, had been losing weight, her coat had lost its shine, and she hadn't come into heat in several years.

In my capacity as staff veterinarian at the Smithsonian National Zoo in Washington, DC, travel to China is part of my job. I like foggy Chengdu, despite the challenges of working in a place where the language and the culture differs so much from mine. And I've gotten into a regular routine when I visit the Panda Base, which houses 35 or so of the world's 260 captive giant pandas. Even so, it's impossible not to feel a bit nervous the night before a scheduled procedure on a giant panda. I know that I'm one of very few veterinarians who will ever have the chance to take care of the animal many people consider the world's rarest and most loved.

I still remember the day in July 1981 when the first living cub was born to a giant panda outside China, at the Chapultepec Zoo in Mexico City. I was twelve years old. A few months later, my mom took my brother, my sister, and me to see the cub, Tohui. We stood in line for almost five hours before reaching the viewing glass that framed the panda's night-house. Because of the great number of people, we were allowed to watch for only a few minutes. We waited anxiously until the mom turned around. Then we saw the fuzzy little black and white baby panda, moving about and trying to climb up his mom's arms. When I saw Ying Ying with her cub, I realized that we were in the presence of an amazing creature. But I never imagined that this exotic species would become a focal point of my career, and indeed of my life.

By the time Tohui turned fourteen, I'd finished veterinary school. That year, the Chapultepec Zoo hired me as staff veterinarian. Working there was a dream come true—the zoo had six giant pandas by then. And yet I wanted to learn more. Unfortunately, no program in my country could offer me further training in zoo animal medicine. Though it was a difficult decision, I decided to leave Mexico in order to become a better veterinarian. I moved to London to do my master's at the Royal Veterinary College under a full scholarship from the British government. Next came a three-year zoo medicine residency at the National Zoo.

Washington's favorite old panda, Hsing Hsing, had just died when I started my program. But two young giant pandas, Mei Xiang and Tian Tian, were on their way from China. Playful and dramatic, they stole the show at the zoo. As in Mexico, people couldn't get enough of watching giant pandas. And they wanted more. So did the zoo staff and its scientists. After some seasons of trial and error, Mei Xiang became pregnant via artificial insemination and gave birth to their first cub, Tai Shan. This was an exciting time for us all, and especially for me: I finished my training that year and was hired by the National Zoo as staff veterinarian, a second dream come true.

On this trip to Chengdu, we planned to examine eight pandas—several with intestinal problems, including Yaloda—over the course of three busy days. Our first day went well. But as we prepared for the next, someone accidentally pushed our endoscope stand. Our fiberscope (a very specialized and expensive piece of equipment) fell to the concrete floor. I reached for it, but wasn't fast enough; as if in slow motion, I watched the delicate instrument land on its base and saw three pieces detach themselves from the lens. A long silence filled the room. No one had to say that we needed the scope tomorrow, when we were scheduled to examine Yaloda.

I evaluated the damage. The piece that attaches the camera to the scope was broken. Without the camera, I could not attach the TV monitor, making it impossible for me to show my Chinese colleagues how to interpret what we'd be seeing inside the panda's stomach and intestines. Nor could I make a recording to document the exam. Without the camera, the scope was virtually useless.

Determined to solve the problem, I gathered my tools: medical tape, scissors, and hair clippers. My improvised fix didn't result in a perfect view through the lens, but it was better than the alternative, which was to cancel the exam on Yaloda. She'd been suffering from some kind of gastrointestinal disease for months. I didn't want her to go any longer without a diagnosis and treatment.

With the key piece of equipment repaired, we reviewed the schedule for the next day: first Yaloda's exam, then two more. We'd start early in the morning, setting up and checking all our equipment, including several plastic crates' worth of veterinary supplies I'd brought from the US. Once everything was ready, each panda would be anesthetized with a combination of drugs injected via a plastic dart.

I also made a point of running through the techniques we'd be using for the endoscopy. Every time we do this procedure together, the Chinese veterinarians gain confidence in their knowledge; one day, they will perform it themselves. When it was safe to handle the panda, we'd move it from its nighthouse to a room with an operating table. We'd insert a tube into its windpipe to protect its airways and place a catheter in one of its arm veins to give it some fluids while under anesthesia. The exam would include an oral exam, abdominal palpation, a blood sample, and endoscopy. This last procedure would be performed with our special, now-repaired fiberscope. We'd introduce the endoscope inside the stomach (gastroscopy) and into the colon of the animal (colono-scopy). Each exam would take two and a half to three hours at least, maybe longer for Yaloda, since we knew she was the panda with the most severe problem.

The night before Yaloda's exam, our excellent hosts took us out to a restaurant, where we ate many colorful, delicious dishes. I felt completely at ease with my Chinese colleagues. Though most of China's traditions are very different from Mexico's, some things are the same. For one thing, Sichuan food is spicy, just like Mexican food. And as at home, friendship and trust are established here over a social meal—socializing that usually includes drinking the traditional Chinese liquor, unless you're doing giant panda anesthesia the next morning! (We had tea, instead.) Chinese *baijou* is very strong, not unlike Mexican tequila. We all looked forward to a proper banquet at the end of our three-day stint.

The next morning, I awoke to the sound of Chengdu's in-cessantly honking cars, a brutal alarm system, and took a taxi to the Panda Base. Before we anesthetize our patients, we like to look at them first. So I found the head veterinarian and we went together to see Yaloda. She was in her night-house, sit-ting on a wooden platform surrounded by stalks of bamboo and piles of loose leaves. It didn't appear as if she'd eaten any-thing overnight. The room temperature was comfortably cool in spite of the heat outside; still, Yaloda seemed uncom-fortable. I could see that her feces were soft.

The panda was thin, her abdomen appeared slightly bloated, and her coat looked dull and coarse. Though only eight years old, she looked older. I'd been told that her feces had been abnormally soft for several years now, and that she had not responded to conventional therapy. In China, "conventional" therapy can vary from traditional Chinese medicine to powerful antibiotics. Although I didn't know why she had not responded to previous treatment, I felt confident that if we could make a definitive diagnosis, we could propose a different treatment and possibly cure her.

Our team had agreed we'd need to perform a colonoscopy on Yaloda as well as gastroscopy. We didn't know for certain which part of her intestinal tract was affected. We'd take small pieces of her stomach and large intestine to be evaluated under the microscope. We hoped this procedure would explain why she'd been sick for such a long time.

Yaloda is a gentle animal, and she was calm before her procedure. When one of the Panda Base vets darted her with the anesthetic drug, she jumped slightly, but then sat back down and watched all of us with her mild dark eyes. I had the impression that she knew that we wanted to help her. I'm sure she found it strange to have so many people paying her all this attention. She fell asleep slowly, having experienced a smooth induction, and continued to do well under anesthesia.

Although I still worried that the scope might break in the middle of the procedure, I felt we had no option—we had to try.

With Yaloda sleeping deeply on her side, we placed a mouth gag between her canines to avoid the possibility of her jaws crushing our scope. I passed the scope in slowly, first into the back of her throat, then down into her esophagus and into the stomach. With the camera and TV monitor running, we could all evaluate the images. Nothing in her

stomach looked abnormal. We decided not to take any biop-
sies there but to move on to the colon. I pulled the scope out
of her mouth and went around to the other end. So far, we'd
found no explanation for her illness. The puzzle was still unsolved.

As soon as we had a clear view of the inside of Yaloda's
large intestine, we could see that the lining, or mucosa, looked
unhealthy, even angry. It was irregular and dotted with red
where it should have been smooth pink. We had our answer.
We took multiple tiny samples of the mucosa—a procedure
used routinely in human medicine—and checked them
under the microscope. As expected, we found severe inflamm-
mation in the cells of the intestinal lining consistent with
inflammation of the colon. Based on these findings, we proposed treatment with a specific medication combining anti-
inflammatory and antibiotic drugs.

Yaloda would likely need this treatment for life. Since
pandas have a life expectancy of twenty-five to thirty years,
this would mean another twenty years or so of treatment. I
was concerned about how she'd tolerate the medication.
Giant pandas can be picky about foods with medicine in
them, and digestive side effects are always possible. We offered Yaloda the medicine in a piece of apple; to my surprise
and relief, she had no problem with it. Indeed, she has turned
out to be a great patient, taking all her meds since day one.
Almost immediately, her intestinal problems started to improve, and soon the consistency of her stool turned normal.

On my next visit to Chengdu, I went to see Yaloda first. She
had gained weight, and her coat was thick and lustrous.
She seemed a happier panda, more energetic and active. She

appeared comfortable this time, even playful. Then, for the first time in many years, Yaloda presented a breeding cycle. Because she'd been so ill, her estrus cycle had been abnormal and the staff at the breeding center had felt she was not a good candidate for pregnancy. Now that she's healthy, Yaloda has been artificially inseminated, a process similar to that performed in humans. We hope Yaloda will become a mom in the near future.

Personally, I couldn't be happier. I had the opportunity to help restore a gentle creature to health, and maybe contribute to the conservation of this rare species if Yaloda is able to have babies. Giant pandas are on loan to zoos around the world, where they receive excellent veterinary care, but there is something very special about working on them in their own land. I look forward to future trips to Chengdu to visit all my friends there—including, of course, Yaloda.

ABOUT THE AUTHOR

Carlos R. Sanchez received his veterinary degree from the National Autonomous University of Mexico (UNAM) in Mexico City. He worked as a veterinarian for Mexico's national zoo, Chapultepec Zoo, from 1992 to 1997. A full scholarship from the British government took him to the Royal Veterinary College in London, where he earned a master's degree in wild-animal health. On his return to Mexico, he worked briefly for the Zoological Society of Mexico and then moved to the United States in 2000 as the first Latin American veterinarian to be accepted in a zoological medicine residency. Dr. Sanchez finished his residency at the Smithsonian National Zoo in 2003 and continued there as a member of the veterinary staff. His current interests include clinical research in anesthesia and the training of Latin American veterinarians, activities that have introduced him to new places and nurtured new friendships. He has published in several veterinary journals and is the co-chair of the International Committee of the American Association of Zoo Veterinarians.

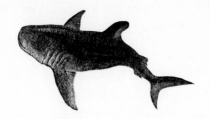

When Whale Sharks Fly

by Howard Krum, MS, VMD, MA

Someone yelled, "The shark is STUCK!"

I blurted out, "What the hell do you mean, the shark is stuck?" Though I was well aware that good veterinarians were expected to be calm, cool, and collected—virtual pillars of medical confidence—my nerves were shot.

The big guy next to me gestured down at one of the high-pressure air casters levitating the 25,000-pound fiberglass box filled with shark and water. "We're stuck," he repeated. The device was jammed on a microscopic crack in the brand-new concrete floor.

I groaned. "Holy crap—you've got to be kidding me."

We were only a few feet, twenty-seven to be exact, from our final destination. We'd just traveled eight thousand miles with two enormous animals code-named "Ralph" and

"Norton" and now were stalled directly in front of our goal. The behemoths were to be the crown jewels for the grand opening of the Georgia Aquarium's brand-new, 6.2-million-gallon Open Ocean exhibit: the world's largest fish tank. The new exhibit was scheduled to open later that year, in November 2005. But at this moment, these two sharks, each well over one thousand pounds, thrashed impatiently in their custom transport containers. The sooner we could release them into the big tank, the better. Just then, Norton regurgitated massively, critically fouling his water—again.

This day had begun over fifty-four hours earlier. Feeling weak, I thought: *I don't handle crises well, or novel challenges, or getting up early in the morning. Why did I take this job?* I am a "big-boned" junk-food connoisseur with the physical vigor of a three-toed sloth, and this marathon mission had required a game plan of outrageous, nail-biting, even death-defying logistics. Why had I signed on for the record-setting transport of two huge whale sharks halfway around the world?

—

Three days earlier, I'd been in Taipei, meeting with the National Fisheries Council. The entire project was on the brink of collapse.

"No, we won't sign it!" said the minister of Taiwanese Fisheries as he slammed his notebook shut, stood up, and began pulling on his jacket. The "it" to which he was referring was a certificate stating, among other things, that the animals would be transported safely and humanely, in accordance with international guidelines. The situation was more than a little ironic, considering that the aquarium had purchased these two animals from a Taiwanese fisherman and they had originally been en route to an Asian dinner table. But without this document, everything would come to a screeching halt: over two years of planning and two hundred million dollars in aquarium construction would be in vain. Moreover, these animals were intended as a surprise gift to the city of Atlanta from Bernie Marcus, our benefactor and the cofounder of The Home Depot.

Our Mandarin-speaking interpreter, Eunice, relayed the rant as the minister and other officials stomped away from the fifty-foot-wide conference table. "Your country insults the Taiwanese government and Taiwan itself! Other countries would not have this requirement."

I grabbed Eunice's hand. "Wait, wait!" I realized that they hadn't understood our request. "Please, sir, this certificate merely states that you believe we are going to transport the animals safely. Your government is certifying *our* efforts, not the other way around."

The fisheries minister paused as the translation sank in. He slowly took off his jacket and returned to the table; so did the twenty-three others.

Dr. Chen, the council's Taipei veterinary representative, spoke next. "Dr. Krum has worked with aquatic animals for years and has brought with him all the supplies the animals could require—medications including IV fluids, medical testing equipment like a blood gas analyzer, an ultrasound unit, and even a water-quality laboratory. He and his team are equipped to deliver better medical care than even humans could receive in flight."

Ten minutes later, they agreed to sign.

On my way out, I shook Dr. Chen's hand gratefully. He said, "I really enjoyed your bluefin tuna presentation at the zoo vets conference in Pittsburgh." *Wow*, I thought, *what a stroke of pure luck.*

From there on out the plan was straightforward: Examine the animals via mask and snorkel to make sure they were fit for flight. On the day of the transport, weather permitting, motor an hour out on two modified ships (one for each animal) to our two-hundred-foot-diameter, fifty-foot-deep sea pen moored off the coast. Then invite the fifteen- and seventeen-foot-long sharks to swim into their stretchers (they'd been trained to do so). Gently crane them on board into temporary, water-filled transport boxes, and head back to the harbor. Lift the animals in custom-made "wet stretchers" (cradling the shark in thousands of gallons of water) and install them in their individual, custom-built ICU transport aquariums with integrated, battery-powered life support. Truck them, us, and approximately five thousand pounds of support gear to the Hualien Airport and load everything onto a heavy-lift prop plane for the short hop to Taipei, where a UPS 747 cargo plane would be waiting. Transfer the animals and take off for Anchorage, where we'd clear customs, get a fresh flight crew, fuel up, and head on to Atlanta. Upon arrival in Atlanta, deplane the boxes onto individual roller-bed tractor-trailers and truck the animals to the aquarium. Offload the enormous boxes onto high-pressure air casters for a short hovercraft ride to the Open Ocean hoist way. Then, with the eight thousand miles and twenty-seven feet behind us, hoist the beasts in their water-filled stretchers up four stories and release them into their spacious new home.

We'd spent months planning every detail of this move. How many other things could go wrong? Compulsively, I'd already run the calculation in my mind: 1,462. None of this—not one single step—had ever been attempted before. And did I mention that the whole plan was to be carried out while flying under the radar of the world press?

As it turned out, the novel challenges had just begun. On the sleepless night before the transport, a sizable earthquake threw me out of bed and onto the floor. This was followed by a thirty-knot gale that miraculously gave way to a sparkling sunrise at sea. Then our sharks inexplicably forgot their training of the past two months. Using buckets of shrimp, we had conditioned them to swim into their stretchers, which they hadn't seemed to mind—until today. Instead, we had to improvise and coax them along with a very big net. Minutes later, Ralph nearly capsized his forty-ton transport vessel when its captain miscalculated the physics of craning the world's largest fish species on board.

Norton's lift went more smoothly. The crane operator on the second, forty-five-foot Chinese fishing boat scooped the leviathan from the ocean without incident, gently depositing him into the seawater-filled twenty-by-six-foot box on the deck. With Norton came a dazzling, life-filled slice of the western Pacific: half a dozen surprised, skin-hugging remora, a tiny school of shimmering jacks, and a rich assortment of colorful seaweeds. It was my first opportunity to see this massive fish up close. His skin tones ranged from a deep, warm slate gray to vibrant aquamarine, dotted with brilliant white spots. I was mesmerized. This was the opportunity we were hoping to offer millions of viewers very soon.

Few people on earth have ever seen a living, breathing, krill-gulping whale shark. The world's largest shark is also the world's largest fish: this gentle, filter-feeding giant can grow to fifty feet in length. Some sharks do eat people, but not this kind. It works the other way around. The flesh of this fish is known as *tofu sha,* an Asian delicacy. And after cruising the world's oceans for sixty million years, this species is vulnerable to extinction thanks to just a few decades of overfishing. The motivation behind our mission—to put Ralph and Norton on public display in the world's largest aquarium—was to inspire millions to care about whale sharks and engender support for their protection.

As our vessel chugged along at five knots, puffing black diesel smoke, we began plowing into subtle ocean swells. Norton started to ram his previously unblemished, three-foot-wide snout into the white fiberglass wall. Contact with any surface is something these animals probably never encountered in the wild. Norton stiffened, appearing stunned by each successive jolt. I envisioned the deepening trauma as thousands of cells were crushed and exploded. If this abuse kept up, it would lead to open ulcerations that could easily become infected. I had no idea how to manage an open wound on the head of an eternally swimming half-ton shark.

A tiny fisherman, clad in fish-slime—encrusted boxers and a yellowing T-shirt, jumped to my aid. We reached for Norton's snout, trying to hold his mass off the wall. It was futile, of course, but in the process, I noticed that the shark was able to withdraw easily from our touch. I experimented by dipping one hand in the water about a foot from Norton's right eye; he was somehow able to recoil despite the continued roll of the ship. Next, I tried just a finger: he maintained his distance. Within minutes, and with just two fingers, we had Norton hovering safely off the container walls. It appeared that this sensitive, gentle hulk just needed a frame of reference. With our success, the fisherman grinned broadly at me and I returned a relieved thumbs-up, the only Mandarin I knew.

As we approached the pier, I saw to my dismay that it was crawling with reporters. Our cover had been blown. Luckily, our captain didn't appreciate the swarm of uninvited guests either. After a brief skirmish that ended with a cameraman swimming for shore, we loaded the animals into their flight containers on flatbed tractor-trailers and made our way to the airport. Here we ran into another snag, a tense standoff with a machine-gun-laden militia who insisted we wait on the tarmac in the scorching sun for government clearance we already had.

The plane's loadmaster, Jose, gave me more bad news. "Doc, these army jerks told me that we have to load and secure the contents of each of the three trucks separately. One at a time on the runway—load, exit, then bring on the next truck."

Knowing that Jose had previously worked as a bodyguard for a warlord in Uganda, I asked, "Do you think you can persuade them to change their minds?"

Jose bullied his way back through the guards and guns to what must have been the officer in charge. After a lot of arm-waving and angry Spanish, he strode back to me.

"I told him, look, if you want to be the reason these animals die on this runway in front of the world media"—he pointed to the cameras only two hundred yards away—"be my guest!" Grinning, Jose slapped me on the back. "Doc, we can load everything now."

About two hours later, crammed with equipment and supplies, including approximately five hundred pounds of ice melting on top of each animal container, the shiny silver prop plane roared to life. With all the doors open it felt like an enormous convection oven stuck on high. We seemed to taxi for miles before the lumbering craft pivoted, the engines revved, and we were off—well, sort of. The plane shimmied and shook and its wings flexed wildly. As we finally felt the ground slip away, I thought I saw razor wire whiz by the open doorway.

One of our Aussie flight crew appeared, wearing a captain's hat, button-down long-sleeved shirt, navy shorts, and a pair of black high-top Converse sneakers. He said, "I think those bloody sharks weigh more than you guessed. We nearly took out that fence. That would have been a bit of a cock-up."

Yeah, I thought—crashing to a fiery death, pulverized by fifty thousand pounds of gear and shark, would indeed have been a bit of a cock-up. Thankfully, we began our descent ten minutes later and glided gracefully into Taipei without incident.

Once on board the 747 cargo plane provided by UPS, I checked the animals, their water-quality and life-support systems. All appeared stable. I could see Norton's and Ralph's eyes and gills through the transport tank portholes. They appeared calmer, cooler, and quite a bit more collected than I felt.

Liftoff for the really long leg of our journey was impressive. We shot from the runway like a rocket—I'm sure we would have won any 747 drag race. The only problem was that the force from all those extra G's must have caused one of our watertight hatches to pop open. A few minutes after takeoff, the copilot scurried down the ladder into the massive cargo hold and grabbed Chris Schreiber by the shoulders. Chris, an affable, unflappable bear of a man with an ever-present Fred Flintstone five-o'clock shadow, was our veteran shark transporter.

The copilot yelled in his face, "There's water leaking somewhere. We've lost electronic control of temperature and cabin pressure!"

The engine roar was deafening. Chris just shrugged as if to say Okay, I'll figure it out. He quickly secured the hatch and reported back. "It's all fixed. We only lost about fifty gallons."

The copilot said, "Good," and nodded at a pocketknife in his hand. "We'll try to control things manually." Fabulous, I thought. If anything else breaks, like, say one of the engines, I've got a bottle opener in my suitcase, just in case.

I compulsively checked and rechecked the water quality. Sharks and other fishes not only produce huge volumes of fecal matter via the usual route, they also excrete pure ammonia from their gills, which in confined spaces can lethally foul their water. But since the water was sparkling, with no detectable ammonia and a dissolved oxygen (DO) concentration of about 115 percent saturation, we decided to nap in shifts.

Four minutes later Chris shook me awake. "Norton's DO is crashing. It's down to 30 percent; he regurgitated buckets of krill—I can't even see him." Immediately, we shifted to plan B and added four industrial-grade air stones attached to cylinders of pure oxygen. The DO gradually climbed to 32 percent and on up from there. Like Norton, we all began to breathe a little easier.

Chris surmised correctly that the chunks of semidigested microshrimp had clogged the aeration atomizer. He skillfully and quickly cleaned the pumps, changed the life support filters, and, for good measure, replaced several of the sixty-pound deep-cycle batteries. Norton's tail tip, now slightly protruding out of the water, was still rhythmically pulsing, so we knew he was alive. In a few hours, the water had cleared enough so we could see that his eyes were clear. Surprisingly, he looked BAR (bright, alert, and responsive). And a bar was exactly where I was headed after this was all over.

Now in Atlanta, stranded just a few feet from his new home, Norton was in trouble again. The shark hung somewhere in the opaque, brick-colored water he'd just created. Unable to see if he was still breathing, I felt cold sweat streaming from my forehead. I got a whiff of myself: I reeked more than usual.

I barked to no one in particular, "We're not going to lose this animal, not now. We gotta change his water immediately."

Several three-inch hoses appeared almost magically and we quickly flushed in clean, well-oxygenated artificial seawater (this was one of the 1,462 potential problems we'd prepared for). I staggered backward. Though this latest crisis had been averted, we'd lost our forward momentum. The jackhammering air compressor was cut off and the boxful of shark and water groaned as it settled on the cracked concrete floor.

After four hours of failed attempts to budge the shark box, someone suggested we try jacking it up with an obviously undersized forklift. At this point, it was worth a try. The forklift's engine growled and the tines shrieked as they were wedged under the massive container. As the driver eased back on the lift lever, he yelled, "Okay, everybody get back, this could be dangerous."

At first, nothing happened except for a lot of ominous cracking and popping. Then the back of the forklift rose swiftly off the ground. This was one of those situations when you don't think, you just do. Ten of us bigger guys scrambled onto the back of the machine behind the driver. Amazingly, the box levered up as the forklift gradually tilted back to the ground. (Relieved, I felt vindicated in my long-held belief that diets were counterproductive; I can only imagine what might have happened to Norton had I curbed my Twinkie intake as so many had foolishly recommended.)

The rest of the move went like clockwork. Only an hour later, a crowd of visitors stood admiring the sharks as they swam calmly in their new Open Ocean home. To a thunderous round of applause, Norton resumed eating, followed soon by Ralph.

For days afterward, I stood at the back of the exhibit gallery assessing the animals' behavior and eavesdropping on our guests.

A little girl would say to her mother: "Mommy, I want to be a marine biologist!"

A little boy would say to his grandfather: "Papa, I love the ocean. And I love Norton."

Me too, I thought, and *that's* why I do this job.

ABOUT THE AUTHOR

Howard N. Krum was born and raised in the Poconos of northeastern Pennsylvania, spending much of his youth on, around, and under the water—frequently skipping school "just to go fishing." He has practiced veterinary medicine at the National Aquarium in Baltimore and at the New England Aquarium in Boston. At the time of the adventure described in this chapter, Dr. Krum was the chief veterinarian and department head of veterinary services and conservation medicine for the Georgia Aquarium. He is currently the zoo pathology resident at the University of Illinois, College of Veterinary Medicine, working with the Shedd Aquarium and the Brookfield and Lincoln Park zoos in Chicago. In addition to a degree in veterinary medicine from the University of Pennsylvania, Dr. Krum has earned a master of science in physiology from Southern Illinois University and a master of arts in science writing from Johns Hopkins University. He has lived, worked, and traveled throughout western Europe and Southeast Asia.

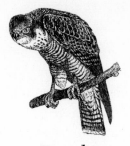

Patch

by Peter Holz, DVSc, MACVSc

As I watched Patch become an ever-smaller speck flying off into the distance, I paused to reflect on his miraculous journey. No doubt it had begun with the screech of tires followed by the inevitable thud and cloud of feathers. Fortunately, someone had found him as he flapped impotently along the roadside, and had the presence of mind to take him to the Healesville Sanctuary veterinary hospital, where he came into my care. The Sanctuary is Australia's largest native fauna park. We do a brisk trade in injured and sick wildlife. That year, 1998, we examined and treated more than fifteen hundred animals that had been smashed by cars, perforated by cats, crunched by dogs, shot, poisoned, and otherwise fallen victim to the planet's current custodians.

My newest patient was a little falcon, also known as a

hobby falcon, one of Australia's smallest birds of prey but no less fierce and proud for his lack of size. He regarded me balefully as I wrapped him in a towel and took him into the examination room. The nurse covered his face with a mask connected to the anesthesia machine, and after several rapid breaths our patient was fast asleep. Now I could examine him without stress. Carefully feeling his wings and shoulders for any abnormalities, I felt a crackling high up on the left side of his body near his neck. We took an X-ray of his wings and body to confirm the diagnosis: the hobby had fractured his coracoid.

The coracoid, a bone absent in mammals, sits high up in the shoulder in birds (part of the "wishbone"). It supports the movement of the wings and helps anchor them to the body. The coracoid is frequently broken by a sudden impact, so we see this type of fracture often in birds, especially raptors that feed near roadways. The trouble is that the coracoid lies submerged beneath a huge slab of breast, or pectoral, muscle— the major muscle group required for flight. These muscles attach to the bone, which acts as a brace. If the coracoid is left to heal on its own, the shoulder joint often stiffens and loses its range of motion.

Because repair requires cutting through these muscles, I had always taken the easy way out. Considering surgery too difficult and also too risky, I had treated prior cases conservatively, prescribing cage rest for a month or so instead. A major reason for the Sanctuary's existence is the treatment and eventual release of injured wildlife. When this is not possible, we are legally required to euthanize the animal. This sounds harsh, but wildlife sanctuaries have limited financial resources and space for injured wildlife. Our mandate is to care for those that have a chance to make it back to the wild. Otherwise, we would soon fill up with crippled animals, denying those with a chance for release the space they need.

Euthanasia was the rule rather than the exception with coracoid fractures in hawks or falcons. The birds recovered but they rarely flew well enough for release. Coracoid fractures were a frustrating and depressing injury for our staff.

My heart sank the moment I saw Patch's X-ray. Yet another bird was doomed. There had to be more I could do for these birds than sticking them in a cage and then killing them a month later. Could surgery be an option? After all, what had I—or, more important, the bird—to lose?

Feeling heroic, I decided that this falcon would be the one. He would live or die by the scalpel, instead of rotting in the cage. The raptor keepers took him to heart and had named him "Patch," after the spot of oddly colored feathers on his chest. This was always a bad omen: naming injured wildlife was an invitation for death to come visit. Just to add to the adrenaline rush, we were in the middle of filming one of those real-life, fly-on-the-wall documentaries. The film crew decided this was an opportunity too good to miss. My first attempt at coracoid surgery would be recorded and shown on national television. The powers that be had already waived their veto rights, allowing the company to film and broadcast anything and everything that they thought would make good TV.

Nowadays it's no big deal to have cameras follow me at work. I operate in a veterinary hospital that exposes every move to the visiting public. But when I took care of Patch, it was all very new and exciting in a terrifying kind of way.

So there I was, with knees trembling and lip wobbling, the bird laid out on the surgery table in front of me, with the skin over his left shoulder area plucked like Sunday's roast chicken to create a sterile field, and the camera perched over my shoulder to capture our triumph or disaster.

The producer wasted no time in taking control of the situation. "Could you move a little to the left, please? You're casting a shadow over the bird. Hold on. Don't start yet, the light isn't right. Could you just put that surgical drape down over the bird again? We'd like to try a different angle this time." The Australian hobby weighs less than eight ounces and the length of its body from head to tail is about ten inches. The people and camera equipment surrounding me made my patient seem even smaller.

Feeling slightly tense, I made my first cut through the skin beside the breastbone and collarbone, and then tentatively delved into the underlying muscle mass. Blood seeped into the wound, but not as much as I had expected. Wherever possible, I tried to separate, or blunt dissect, the muscle fibers rather than cut through them. An alarmingly large grouping, or plexus, of assorted blood vessels and nerves appeared. Though my surgical instruments were deep in the bird's chest, the hole I had made was tiny, like a keyhole, making my frustratingly thick fingers feel even clumsier than usual. No concert pianists in my family.

I felt around for the fracture ends for what seemed like an eternity, conscious of the camera whirring away. Finally I located one end of the broken bone and inserted a metal rod into its cavity, which I drove up and out through the soft tissue of the shoulder. Lining up this end with the other broken bone end, I reversed the pin and pushed it into the bone. I had to be careful. If I pushed too far I would enter the chest cavity and pierce the bird's heart. That would make exciting television. Fortunately, I managed to align the fracture ends successfully, and the pin sat nicely within the bone.

At this point, our senior raptor keeper asked if I would be cutting off the length of pin, which currently protruded from Patch's shoulder. To relieve the tension, I said flippantly, "No, if we leave it sticking out, it will be easier to catch him when he flies past." I still wince when I remember hearing myself say that on national television.

All that was left now was to sew up the butchered muscle and skin. This part of the surgery went quickly. Much to my relief, Patch and I both recovered uneventfully from the procedure. We kept the falcon confined in a small cage to give the bone ends time to knit together. During the initial post-surgical period, he received antibiotics and analgesics in his food. Patch's appetite was good and after three weeks we decided to X-ray his shoulder. Though the alignment of the fracture ends was not perfect, the bone had healed. A bird's higher metabolic rate allows fractures to mend much faster than in a mammal. We removed the pin and Patch entered rehab, much like an injured human athlete.

The raptor keepers devised an exercise regime for Patch, gradually increasing his workload over time. He was initially encouraged to take short flights between perches within a room to see if he could actually maintain height. After mastering this simple exercise, he was moved to a larger aviary with a greater distance between perches. While aviary flight gave us some idea of his capabilities, we needed to build up his fitness and see how well he could maneuver in flight. So we placed leather anklets on his legs that were attached to a long line called a creance. The next step was to allow him to fly free.

This stage of rehabilitation for Patch resembled the methods used by falconers to train their birds to hunt pigeons. The keepers used a food-based reward system to encourage him to return, throwing pieces of pigeon into the air so that he was forced to dive, turn, and attack. They would launch Patch into flight and then bring him back with the food. It was important to test his newly healed bone as thoroughly as possible to ensure that it would withstand the rigors of daily flight in the wild. Patch passed all his tests and slowly gained both strength and fitness. The film crew keenly followed his progress.

After more than three months of hard work, we decided Patch was ready to return to the wild. A convoy of excited keepers and the camera crew drove out to the release site, not far from where the falcon was initially found. We bounced along a rough farm track in our four-wheel drives, coming to a halt under a small grove of trees. Patch's box was removed from the back of my vehicle; a radio transmitter was attached to his tail feathers so that we could track his progress. I was given the honor of releasing Patch, cameras buzzing in the background. He glared at me without a hint of gratitude or recognition and I threw him into the overcast sky.

He flew straight as an arrow, rapidly becoming a tiny speck in the distance. Then he disappeared completely. The steady beep from the radio receiver remained the only evidence of his existence.

We tracked Patch daily for the next two weeks and monitored his progress. Sadly, most animals are released back to the wild with no follow-up. Many rehabilitation facilities either don't have the necessary transmitters or lack the staff for extended monitoring. In such cases, no one knows if all the time and effort expended on the animal has paid off. The Sanctuary has made this last step of rehabilitation a priority. We follow all of our raptors postrelease, which has allowed us to gather detailed information showing that many birds do rehabilitate successfully and survive long term.

In Patch's case, the tracking team established that he was hunting and flying normally. But we couldn't be certain that he was catching enough food to maintain his weight. From a distance, birds can appear strong one day, only to die emaciated the next. So after two weeks we decided to capture him for a final examination. Using a Swedish goshawk trap baited with food, we were able to catch the falcon easily without hurting him.

I examined him there in the middle of a field, holding him in a towel. He seemed decidedly put out to be in my hands again and tried unsuccessfully to bite me. Patch had gained weight since release, a sure sign that he was coping well and finding enough of his own food to survive. We removed the radio transmitter and released him back to the wild for the final time. I watched once again as he took to the air, indistinguishable in flight from any other hobby falcon.

Each journey begins with a single step, and Patch's was the first in my coracoid repair journey. Since that day, I have surgically repaired all coracoid fractures and have taught the technique to both students and veterinarians. Not every case has been as spectacularly successful as Patch's. Even so, we now release into the wild over 90 percent of birds presented with coracoid fractures, making it our most successful avian orthopedic procedure.

Despite all the stress and anxiety, the television piece didn't end up looking too bad, either.

ABOUT THE AUTHOR

Peter Holz graduated from the University of Melbourne veterinary school with first-class honors in 1987. In 1994, he completed a combination degree as doctor of veterinary science in zoo animal medicine and pathology through the University of Guelph in Canada; he became a diplomate of the American College of Zoological Medicine in 1995 and a member of the Australian College of Veterinary Scientists in Medicine of Zoo Animals in 1996. Dr. Holz has been employed at Healesville Sanctuary, Australia's largest native fauna park, since 1994. His major research interests include drug pharmacokinetics in reptiles, orthopedic surgery on and rehabilitation of raptors, coccidiosis in macropods, and—more generally—the impact of disease on Australian wildlife.

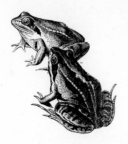

Anesthesia for a Frog

by Mark Stetter, DVM

One of the coolest things about frogs is that they can breathe through their skin. Of all the animals I work with, I think they are my favorite—and for a long time I was frustrated with the existing methods of frog anesthesia. A common technique involved using a powdered fish anesthetic, MS-222, dissolved in a water bath. In fish, it is a very safe and effective method. As the fish swims, the drug becomes absorbed across the gills and into the bloodstream; the patient falls asleep in a couple of minutes and rapidly wakes up when removed from the medicated water. In frogs, this drug is much more slowly absorbed through the skin, requiring as many as thirty minutes to induce anesthesia and a very long time (sometimes hours) for recovery. There is also the fact that many terrestrial frogs dislike being forced to take a long bath in the anesthetic water.

It seemed to me that frogs deserved a better anesthetic protocol, and that the key to this lay in their amazing skin. I wondered if a liquid anesthetic, applied directly, might possibly work.

I continued to ponder the concept until the right opportunity finally arose. At the time (1996), I was working as a veterinarian at the Wildlife Conservation Society's Bronx Zoo in New York City. One day, I was on rounds at our Central Park facility when our curator of reptiles and amphibians approached me and said, "Mark, I need you to look at a frog while you're here this morning. I think there was a big frog rumble in the tank last night, and when I came in this morning one of the frogs looked pretty beat up."

We had our first patient! Frances was an ideal candidate— a beautiful poison dart frog from our new South American rain forest exhibit. She was brightly colored, with alternating markings of vivid blue and black. But although these little frogs seem cute and harmless to us, they can be quite savage toward each other. They often exhibit aggressive behavior in the effort to establish dominance, territory, and breeding rights. Frogs are no different from other animals in this respect.

Poison dart frogs get their name from hunters in South America. Indigenous peoples have long used the toxic excretions from the skin of this species as a fast-acting poison. When the tip of a dart is rubbed on the skin of the frog, the dart becomes a lethal projectile to bring down animals in the forest. Even more interesting, rain forest poison dart frogs do not produce this toxin when housed in zoos and aquariums. Nothing else about the animal changes; a captive frog looks and behaves exactly like a wild one. Scientists think the rain forest frogs ingest the primary components of the toxins via certain wild insects and other foods found only in the jungle—hence their deadly skin.

Somehow, Frances had been injured in the group frog fight, and her left eye appeared to have been punctured. Although she was a fully grown adult, Frances was only the size of a dime, and her eye was about the size of a blunt pencil tip. I would need our surgical microscope to see the extent of the damage and, if possible, repair it—a very delicate procedure. But how could I safely anesthetize her and ensure that she didn't move, not even slightly, while I performed this critical surgery under the microscope?

It was time to try my new frog anesthesia program.

The anesthetic gas called isoflurane is used in people, dogs, cats, horses, and a variety of wildlife species. Purchased as a liquid in a small glass bottle, isoflurane is poured into a metal compartment inside the anesthetic machine. A tank of oxygen is also connected to the machine. When the machine is turned on, it mixes isoflurane with oxygen and forms an anesthetic gas. The usual method of delivering the gas is to place a mask over the patient's face or insert an endotracheal tube in his windpipe (trachea). With frogs, both of these options are difficult, if not impossible. Holding a tiny face mask over the nose of a small, slippery frog is not an easy task. (I know, I've tried it.)

If frogs can breathe through their skin, why can't we just apply the isoflurane directly on their skin?

I knew from my previous work that you can place the entire frog in a mask, creating a little frog anesthetic chamber, and the frog will eventually fall asleep. The problem with the frog chamber is that it takes a very long time for the anesthesia to be effective.

Frogs can also be directly injected with anesthetic, like any mammal, but the effects are variable and the dose difficult to measure. If too little is given, the patient will move, making delicate surgery impossible. If too much is given, it's lethal. In a patient this small, even with the world's smallest syringe and a lot of drug dilution, injectable anesthetic was neither safe nor practical.

If I could succeed in applying the liquid isoflurane directly to the frog's skin, I'd not only be able to avoid the prolonged anesthetic gas chamber method, I'd also be developing a technique that could be used anywhere. Researchers could utilize this method for sedating amphibians in the field; it could also be used by zoo and aquarium vets in countries that might not have access to expensive anesthetic machines.

Liquid isoflurane is very volatile, so much so that a single drop evaporates in a matter of seconds. I knew that I'd need to mix the liquid anesthesia with something that would slow the evaporation rate and allow greater time for the anesthetic drug to be absorbed through the frog's skin.

I decided to combine the liquid isoflurane with water and a type of skin lubricant, K-Y Jelly, to create an elixir. I mixed the ingredients into a thick, syrupy solution that could be gently applied to our frog, calculating that the jelly would slow the rate of evaporation.

I applied a couple of drops to Frances's back, then placed

her in a small clear plastic container. I pulled my chair up to the surgery table and waited. Within a couple of minutes, I could see the drug starting to take effect. Frances was getting a little woozy and was swaying from side to side. It was work-ing! But would she become anesthetized enough so that the surgery could be performed? And if so, for how long would the two drops work?

After about five minutes, Frances could not sit upright; she rolled onto her side, sound asleep. I waited a couple of minutes longer and then removed her from the container for a full anesthetic check. In a frog, a "full anesthetic check" isn't performed with fancy EKGs, stethoscopes, or pulse oxime-ters. In even the tiniest frogs like Frances, you can actually see the heart beating beneath the skin. She had a good heart-beat, there was no movement, and when I pinched her tiny little toe there was no response. Perfect!

Off to surgery she went. Even with the surgical micro-scope, this was going to be a challenge. I had our veterinary intern scrub in with me to maximize the chance of success. When performing microsurgery, it's important to keep your eyes focused on the image in the microscope. You don't want to look up for any reason, and your elbows need to stay planted on the table. Your assistant is in charge of exchanging the surgical instruments in your hand.

Operating microscopes are commonly used for eye surgery in both humans and animals, particularly for cataract removal. This type of delicate procedure requires magnifica-tion for the surgeon and a complete lack of eye movement from the patient. Even a partial eyelid blink can be disas-trous. In Frances's case, I was not only concerned about movement, I also knew we'd be pushing the limits of the microscope, designed for work on human-size eyes. Our entire patient was smaller than a human eye!

Examination under the microscope confirmed the damage: Frances's eye had been ruptured, and she was not going to be able to see out of it again. At this point, our only hope was to save her eye and minimize the chance for infection. Bacteria or fungal organisms could infect the eye, spread throughout her body, and jeopardize her life. We used the smallest type of suture material available to place a single stitch through her cornea. Usually a corneal laceration would require several sutures to repair, but in this small patient, only one was needed.

It took Frances about thirty minutes to wake up from the anesthesia. This was a good indicator that I had used the correct amount of anesthetic to begin with. After the surgery, she spent the night in the hospital's frog ICU—a warm, moist, quiet, well-monitored plastic container. The next day, she went back to the rain forest building for close observation.

I'd been concerned that Frances might need additional surgeries and that we would be forced to remove the eye altogether. But when I made a house call to check the frog in her exhibit a couple of days later, it was obvious she was going to heal well. The tissue of the injured eye looked healthy and she did not appear overly bothered by either the injury or the surgery. The keepers had helped her find her food and given her some extra attention after she returned from the hospital.

In the wild, frogs need both of their eyes to feed. They

have exceptional vision, which they use in their aggressive capture of flying insects. Now Frances would need help catching her food on a long-term basis. To give her a competitive edge, the zookeepers found a way to slow down the live insects: they chilled them. By placing the food in the refrigerator prior to mealtime, they could slow the insects' flight, allowing Frances to get her necessary food requirements.

Since that day with Frances, I have used the topical isoflurane jelly protocol with many frogs and toads. By presenting this method of amphibian anesthesia at various scientific meetings and writing about it for veterinary medical books, I have also shared this technique widely with my colleagues. But it was Frances, our tiny poison dart frog, that made it all happen.

ABOUT THE AUTHOR

Mark D. Stetter received his bachelor's degree in biochemistry and chemistry, followed by a veterinary degree from the University of Illinois at Urbana–Champagne. He completed an internship in small animal medicine and surgery at the Animal Medical Center in New York and then served as staff veterinarian at the Audubon Institute in New Orleans. Dr. Stetter went on to complete a residency in zoological medicine at the Bronx Zoo / Wildlife Conservation Society, where he became associate veterinarian. He joined Disney's Animal Kingdom in 1997, when it first opened, and is currently director of veterinary services. He is board certified by the American College of Zoological Medicine, serving as president of this organization in 2006–2007. Known among his friends and colleagues for thinking outside the box, Dr. Stetter has a special interest in medical technology and has been the first to apply advanced diagnostic and treatment techniques in a wide range of species, from frogs to elephants.

III

GETTING PHYSICAL

Zoo vets face unique challenges because of the vast number of species in their care, the potentially endless list of medical problems, and the great variety of conditions in which wild animals live. They must be prepared to be emergency doctors, primary caregivers, anesthesiologists, surgeons, even gerontologists. Every day is different, and many cases are one of a kind. The work can be exhausting, uncomfortable, and dangerous.

We begin our examination of every patient with what sounds like a simple process: observation. Since most wild animals have an innate fear of humans, even this first step can be hard on the doctor. In field situations, we may track the patient for hours or even days before we catch a glimpse of it. If the animal has learned to recognize the vet, we may end up hiding in vehicles, climbing trees, or sitting motionless at a distance until the animal accepts and ignores our presence. Sometimes the only option may be to join the animal in its environment: plenty of zoo vets have donned a wet suit and scuba gear and swum with their patients, even with sharks.

Once we decide it's necessary to restrain, anesthetize, or move a wild animal, we plan our approach. These procedures may carry a certain degree of risk, depending on the animal and the circumstances. Whereas an inch-long Texas dung beetle can be held gently in a pair of forceps, a 250-pound tiger requires a carefully placed anesthetic dart. Human safety is always a top priority. And even with the best planning, anything can happen.

If we don't have personal experience with the particular animal or situation—always a possibility—we review what we've done with closely related animals, read the literature, and call for advice.

Many smaller birds, reptiles, amphibians, and invertebrates can be carefully held in a net or in gloved hands. To minimize stress, it's best to lightly anesthetize them for an exam. But larger species that can bite, kick, scratch, and expel venom must be immobilized from the start. In such cases, we use a variety of potent injectable anesthetics in addition to gas anesthesia. Sometimes these drugs can be injected by hand, with the animal in a net or restraint box. More often, we inject them from a distance by a flying dart, using a lightweight CO_2-powered pistol or rifle.

Zoo vets tend to work long hours in difficult settings, whether it's kneeling on a concrete floor performing surgery or crawling through brambles to see a patient. Even a state-of-the-art veterinary hospital can feel like the bush when you've been working for sixteen hours every day for a week. When we work in the field, whether easily accessible or remote, all of the necessary equipment and staff must be brought to the patients. Checklists are essential, given that something unpredictable always happens. Most of us subscribe to the rule that says plan, plan, plan . . . and then be flexible.

Zoo vets are known for their stamina, strong constitutions, steady hands, good aim, and healthy knees—with a bit of ego added to the mix. In this next selection of stories, these vets get physical. One works nonstop for a solid month to fly a group of dolphins to a new home. Another takes a risk while examining one of the world's largest saltwater crocodiles. Others brave logistical challenges and harsh conditions before they even have a chance to get their hands on their patients—a Bactrian camel, a herd of escaped bison, a mountain gorilla, and a forest elephant.

Lucy H. Spelman, DVM

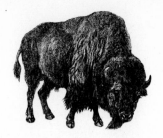

La Recapture (The Recapture)

by Florence Ollivet-Courtois, DVM

I've never been successful anesthetizing a bison. Are you sure?" Over the phone, the owner of the herd sounded both demanding and doubtful. He too was a veterinarian. "The smallest animal weighs at least seven hundred kilograms and most weigh well above one thousand kilograms." He gave me this information as if I'd never even seen a bison.

A few days earlier, I'd heard on the news that the French Army planned to shoot and kill an entire herd of escaped bison if something wasn't done soon. For the past three weeks, the animals had been wandering around the French countryside near the farm where they lived in the village of Joinville. TV crews had filmed them: the large, shaggy brown animals with huge horns appeared to be enjoying their freedom, trampling crops, eating what they liked, and charging through small villages. It was the end of May 2004; maybe they decided the grass looked better on the other side of the fence. The authorities had tried to capture them with dogs and horses but succeeded only in running the herd around even more. Now they planned to use bullets.

I vowed not to let that happen. I felt confident that a full-scale bison recapture was achievable, especially with the help of my husband, Marc, a fire-and-rescue official who also knows how to handle scared or injured animals.

"I've used Immobilon numerous times to anesthetize rhinos, elephants, and bison, including big, excited animals," I replied. "I've got enough of this drug for twenty animals, more than half your herd. We can do this."

A highly potent narcotic, Immobilon is a controlled drug, and there are strict laws about its use. We have to pay for a special license to use this anesthetic on animals and are required to keep a detailed log that accounts for every drop. Only a few companies sell this drug, or a similar one; it must be imported into France from the UK; and we can only buy so much at once. But although I didn't have enough of this anesthetic for the entire herd of thirty-plus animals, I knew that bison always travel together. If we moved some, the others would follow.

With his reluctant acquiescence, I directed the owner of the bison herd to prepare for our arrival. He would need several tractor-trailers equipped with some type of lift in order to raise the anesthetized animals off the ground and transport them.

I learned that the situation had indeed become critical. As the big animals smashed down fences, they inadvertently set hundreds of cows free as well. Farmers struggled to keep up with repairs and round up their cows. They were angry. A ranger with a rifle had managed to reduce the herd by one, shooting a bison that charged a village crowd. But when the officials proposed shooting all of the animals, the general public and animal-welfare groups reacted with outrage. In any case, this option was not only unacceptable, it was also impractical. The bison would certainly disperse at the sound of gunshots.

Finally, acting on the advice of the rangers' office and the director of the Paris Zoo, where I used to work, the veterinarian who owned the bison herd called me. He had run out of choices.

The following afternoon, Marc and I flew to eastern France. Our equipment included an unusual assortment of gear, and we were relieved when the French airport authorities cleared us through security. Most people traveling with rifles, drugs, ropes, and heavy leather straps would not get very far at Paris Charles de Gaulle International Airport!

After an hour's flight, we were met by a local government official and driven by truck to the section of countryside where the escaped bison had been grazing for the past week. Using a pair of powerful binoculars high on a hill, I watched the herd moving about peacefully in the middle of a field dotted with spring flowers—and noticeably empty of cows. Several bison drank water from a tank. Others rested lying down. The fugitives looked completely calm.

About two dozen frustrated farmers had gathered for the capture event. They regarded me warily. The veterinarian who owned the herd stood silent in the middle of the crowd.

The bison had pushed through or trampled every fence in their path, forcing the farmers to round up their cattle and lock them in barns. I could see that managing the people during this event would be half the challenge, so I began with a detailed briefing to explain a number of precautions.

"The anesthetic we use for the bison, Immobilon, is designed for large-animal anesthesia and is very dangerous to humans. It has two great advantages: potency and reversibility. A tiny amount fells a bison in less than ten minutes. Its full effect will last only an hour, but the animal will remain heavily sedated unless the drug is reversed. We carry an antidote that completely antagonizes the narcotic and can return the animal to its feet in minutes."

I went on to explain the disadvantage: while this anesthetic is safe for hoofed animals like bison, giraffes, rhinos, and gazelles, just two drops on the skin or splattered in the eye or mouth will kill a person in less than five minutes. It is quickly absorbed and shuts down the respiratory system.

Because of this danger, I asked that everyone give us plenty of room to maneuver. Though the antidote does work on people, I emphasized that our goal was to avoid any situation in which we'd have to use it. No one should touch the darts or the animals when they first fell down under the effects of the anesthetic. Marc and I would remove the dart and pick up any that missed their targets. Helpers should avoid getting any blood from the animals on their hands. (Theoretically, the drug poses no risk to humans once it's in the bison's bloodstream, but I did not want to put this theory to the test.)

Next I explained the risks to the animal. Anesthesia in bison is risky because they tend to vomit. Moving the animals can accentuate this tendency, since their normal reflexes are disabled by the anesthetic. The material in the rumen, the fermentation-vat portion of the stomach, includes a mixture of plant fiber, fluid, and gas. If the bison vomits under anesthesia, this material practically explodes out of the animal's mouth. It's usually impossible to clear it away from the area over the back of the tongue fast enough to prevent it from ending up in the wrong place—the opening to the airway.

I emphasized that the way to minimize this possibility was to keep the animal's head above its belly at all times. Everyone needed to follow this rule. Marc would place a sling around the bison's body and use a tractor with a pitchfork-style front-end loader to raise the animal off the ground. After looping the sling around the metal tines, Marc would ask for help in holding the bison's head up while its body was lifted into the trailer. This could take two additional people, given the size of the animals.

The farmers appeared to be listening, though several smiled or raised their eyebrows. After all, they'd been trying to capture the bison for weeks, without success. How could a woman from the city do better in one day? It also occurred to me that they might not mind if a bison or two died after all the damage the animals had caused. But I did mind.

I closed the briefing with a question: "Does anyone know if it's possible to drive a truck past the herd without disturbing them?" The farmers answered yes, no problem. We could proceed as planned.

Marc and I climbed into the truck, each armed with a loaded dart rifle and a second dart at the ready. We both wore dark green coveralls and latex rubber gloves. I had my stethoscope in my pocket as well as the reversal drug already drawn up in a capped syringe, just in case. Each animal would receive the same dosage of Immobilon, 1.5 milliliters. Despite the stress of the situation, I felt a rush of adrenaline. I loved working with Marc, and was determined to save these roving bison.

In case one of the bison charged the truck, a ranger with a bullet rifle accompanied us as a precaution. We drove toward the herd. The animals seemed oblivious. I fired the first dart from about forty meters, into the rear end of a large female to the right of the truck. Marc got his dart off a minute later, into the shoulder of a male on the left.

Thanks to their tough hides, both bison reacted as if stung by a bee rather than a dart. They barely moved, and the herd stayed together. We reloaded and darted again. Ten minutes from the start, we had darts in four animals. They began to react, staggering and then slumping to the ground. The other bison continued to rest or eat, seemingly unperturbed.

With the herd still so calm, I decided we should dart another group before moving the first animals to the trailers. Once we began to work on the anesthetized bison, the others would figure out that something scary was happening. Marc and I loaded our darts again, and drove back past the group of bison. Within another ten minutes, we'd anesthetized four more bison. Of the thirty-five escapees, we already had eight under control. I glanced over at the group of farmers. Their expressions had changed dramatically. They looked astonished.

We approached the eight sleeping bison one by one, removing the darts and checking their breathing. As expected, the rest of the herd ran off, but they didn't go far. Most remained in the thick bush on the edge of the clearing. Marc and the farmers repositioned several of the anesthetized animals, rolling them into a sternal position with their legs under them and their heads propped up on a block of wood or on the farmer's knees. This helped them breathe more easily and reduced the risk of vomiting.

In an ideal setting, we would have taken the time to monitor blood oxygen levels, and maybe even secure an airway by passing a tube down the windpipe. But with limited resources and so many animals to dart, our plan was to get them down and up again as soon as possible. The longer bison remain under anesthesia, the more likely they'll bring up food material.

I gave each bison a physical exam and collected blood samples while Marc readied them for the move. He tied their front and rear legs together with ropes in preparation for hooking them up to a sling.

In his enthusiasm, the veterinarian-owner forgot my earlier advice. I turned to see him running the tractor's controls, lifting a female bison by a rope looped around the pitchfork loader and tied to a single forelimb, as if she were a dead cow. My heart sank. When he put her down on the flatbed trailer, she vomited copious amounts of watery, fibrous green material. I knew instantly we couldn't save her.

The female died from suffocation seconds later. I'm afraid I lost my temper, shouting, *"Faites chier! C'est pas la peine de se casser le cul à vous expliquer si vous foutez tout en l'air!"* Translation (minus the curse): "I took great pains to take the time to explain what to do and you still screwed up!"

Marc kept his calm. He showed the veterinarian how to place the sling so it would support the bison's entire body, rather than raise just one limb. He placed the main straps first: one under the animal's belly, one behind the front legs, and the other just in front of the rear legs. Then he looped two smaller straps around the neck and tail, linking these to the main sling. After checking all the connections, Marc hooked the two main straps onto the tractor's pitchfork and directed the farmer to raise it slowly. Gradually the bison's body rose about three feet off the ground, just high enough to be moved onto the trailer. All the while, two people held on to the bison's head to keep it elevated above its belly.

Within an hour after we'd fired our first darts, seven bison were lying in a row in the trailer. We gave the antidote to each one, and they recovered to a standing position minutes later. Several farmers hauled the dead bison away, with strict instructions to incinerate the body. The narcotic anesthetic would still be in the animal's system. The meat could not be safely consumed by anyone—human or animal.

We reloaded and continued darting, though now our work was more difficult. We had to approach the remaining animals slowly, and the darts upset the herd this time. Several darted animals ran off, three of them falling asleep in the woods. We found ourselves struggling through brambles to reach them. We had to manhandle several bison into the clear before we could use the tractor's pitchfork and trailer. But thanks to the large group of farmers on hand, we managed to move them all safely.

By midday, we'd anesthetized eighteen bison. Marc and I had concentrated on darting the dominant animals, as well as the largest and most dangerous ones. We planned to move the group of eighteen to the owner's barn, several kilometers away. Bison behave just like cows—or giraffes, for that matter: they are highly social. We predicted that the other sixteen herd members would long for their companions and follow on their own. The farmers questioned this plan, while the owner wanted us to continue with the anesthesia. Either he'd forgotten or did not want to believe that I only had enough of the special drug for half the herd.

The recaptured bison called for their companions all night. By the next day, the remaining herd had found their way back to the bison barn. Just a few hours later, one of the females even gave birth to a healthy calf. The veterinarian-owner never directly thanked us, but he did show his appreciation by naming the calf "Essonne," after the French state where Marc and I live.

Back home in Paris that night, we switched on the TV to watch the evening news. This time, the story began with "The thirty-five escaped bison are back in their enclosure. A special team from Paris got the better of the bison's thirst for freedom." I watched my interview. The reporter wanted to know if the situation was dangerous. "Yes," I told him, "but everything went fine, thanks to the help of everybody involved: farmers, authorities, and veterinarians."

In France, the meat of an animal anesthetized with Immobilon at any point during its lifetime can never be consumed. As a result, the herd lives on. We saved them not once but twice!

ABOUT THE AUTHOR

Florence Ollivet-Courtois comes from a family of veterinarians, representing the fourth generation to take up the profession. She earned her veterinary degree from the Alfort Veterinary School in Paris, and has worked on the staff of the Paris Zoo (Musée National d'Histoire Naturelle) for eight years, currently serving as a veterinary consultant in zoo and wildlife medicine and surgery. She is a consultant for sixteen European zoos—and volunteers in a firefighter department in a southern suburb of Paris, where her husband, Marc, a professional firefighter, specializes in rescue-dog training and dangerous-animal capture. Dr. Ollivet-Courtois is a member of the European Association of Zoo and Wildlife Veterinarians and the French Association of Zoo Veterinarians. Her areas of expertise include large animal anesthesia, wild animal transport, and zoo renovation. She is in charge of the veterinary aspects of the brown bear reintroduction program in southern France.

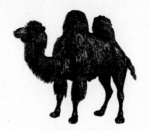

A Camel in the Snow

by Christian Walzer, DVM

My numbed mind is trying to determine if the sun has risen. Do I really have to get up? The daily battle between sleep, a full bladder, and the misery of leaving my warm sleeping bag for the cold outside begins anew. But the day's work awaits. Maybe we'll capture our first wild camel.

Our small team—myself; Petra, my biologist colleague and research partner; and a half dozen others—has been camping in Mongolia's Gobi Desert since the beginning of November (2005). It's been three weeks and we've yet to see a Bactrian (two-humped) camel. With only about five hundred remaining in the wild, they are among the rarest animals in the world. And we know very little about them. Our mission is to capture three Bactrian camels and outfit them with high-tech satellite collars that will allow us to track their movements. The data produced by our research will contribute to the development of a conservation action plan for this critically endangered species.

Through the tiny open slit of my sleeping bag, I see the immobile shape of Petra. Apparently she's still asleep, or at least pretending. With my toes, I can feel the boxes of drugs, batteries, and other objects stored inside my sleeping bag; my body heat protects them from the low temperatures.

Eventually, as it does every morning, my bladder wins. I crawl out of the bag and get showered by ice crystals. They form each night on the inside surface of the tent, frozen remnants of the moisture contained in our respirations. I look around for my clothes. At −25° centigrade (−13° Fahrenheit), getting dressed is a daily trial. I hold my breath, telling myself this is not the time to wimp out, and slip my feet into my rock-hard frozen boots. I pull the tent zip up and poke my head out. Gerelmaa is already up and has a fire going to melt snow for tea and coffee. She calls out, *"Sain bainuu?"*—the all-purpose ritual greeting in Mongolia.

"Sain bainaa, I'm fine!" I answer back.

With the first hot mug of milk tea in my hands and the warming fire, the world looks and feels a better place already. A great white expanse of snow surrounds us. Not a single tree interrupts the view. In the distance, rolling hills and mountains with sharp-edged dark rocks catch the first pink rays of sunlight. Rivulets of wind-driven ice crystals flow around the campsite like small streams. Our three hobbled domestic camels watch impassively as the camp awakens. I've journeyed to this area several times a year for nearly ten years. Even so, I am in awe of the Gobi this morning.

We've been traveling through the very remote southern part of the Gobi Desert, one of the world's great desert ecosystems. The extremely harsh environment has given rise to unique and particularly well-adapted species, many of which are found nowhere else in the world. Among them is the wild Bactrian camel, the fine-boned ancestor of the domestic camel we so often see in zoos. Thousands of Bactrian camels once roamed this region. Though they now live in a protected area, their population has steadily declined, primarily due to human encroachment on their fragile home.

It took us two weeks just to get to the desert. After a further frustrating week inside the protected area, we have yet to see a single camel. Now we are just 37 miles north of the Chinese border fence.

Petra is up. She walks over to the fire sleepily, looking for her mug. "Morning. Is Adiya already looking for camels?"

"I saw him on the ridge earlier with the spotting scope," I reply. "Let's keep our fingers crossed." Petra puts a frozen slab of bread on a shovel and pushes it into the fire to make some toast. Suddenly the radio spurts to life. Tumaa, our driver and park ranger, is quick to get the call. *"Tsaa, Tsaa bainuu!"* It's Adiya, calling in from the ridge. I can't understand most of what he says, but between the cacophonic garbling I pick up the words *"khavgai, khavgai"*—wild camel.

Finally, after a long week of searching, we have our first sighting. Immediately, I begin to feel the excitement of the chase. Our trusty Russian UAZ-model jeeps are still frozen, however. They'll need a fire under the gearbox and both axles before we can move out. The team is quick to mobilize. Tumaa starts two blowtorches under the jeep and removes the window on the passenger side so that I'll be able to get a good shot with the dart gun.

Getting the darts ready is a long and delicate procedure. For this capture, we use a novel drug combination that includes five individual components. The most important of these is the opiate etorphine, an extremely potent wildlife capture drug similiar to Immobilon. Though a few drops can potentially kill a human, it's a great drug for the anesthesia of large mammals. Thanks to the cold, all of the drugs have to be thawed and then laced with sterile antifreeze. I do this carefully—and slowly. It's a struggle to work the syringes with precision; my fingers feel numb inside my thick gloves. Petra keeps a close eye on me, just in case I jab myself with the dangerous mix. I finally get four darts ready, cap each needle with a protective cover, and place them inside my down jacket, close to my body to keep them from freezing solid.

"Okay, let's get going," I call out to the others. "We don't want to lose them again."

The team crawls into the jeeps. We make one last check that we have everything we need, and off we go. Even though I am wearing several layers of clothes and a full-face mask, the stinging cold air rushing in through the open window frame takes my breath away. But not for long. The chase is on, and absolutely everything else forgotten.

The jeep carefully inches up toward the ridge. We don't want the camels to pick us out against the skyline. Adiya and I jump out and crawl up to the rim. There, below us, is a herd of twenty-five camels moving calmly up the valley in search of something to eat. Every now and then, one of them lifts its head and has a look around. Not seeing anything out of the ordinary, the head drops again.

Most of the camels are females and juveniles, but at the edge of the group is a very large male camel. "Look at him," Adiya whispers. "He's really big. What a beautiful animal!"

I whisper back, "I think we should try for this bull. The terrain over to the east is flat and looks quite easy for a chase by jeep. A surprisingly good approach." We carefully slide back down out of sight.

To the extent that our old jeep can actually attain significant speed, Tumaa has the vehicle flying over the ridge. The camels see us and freeze momentarily. Then they start running along the valley in their typical pacing gait. Their bodies lengthen as they gather momentum, the front and rear legs on each side reaching forward and backward in perfect synchrony.

"All right, let's go! Tumaa, get the jeep behind the bull. Over there!" I yell over the whining engine noise. Ever so slowly, the bull gets larger. I raise the dart gun and begin to focus through the scope. The camel appears in the scope and is instantly gone again as we hit the next bump.

"Tumaa, we must get a bit closer. . . . Looks good." I have the bull clearly in the scope and think, *Relax, don't shoot too soon—just wait, wait.* For a brief moment the motion of the jeep seems suspended and I pull the trigger. With a distinct *swoosh,* the compressed carbon dioxide pushes the dart down the barrel. Time slows, and through the scope I watch the dart streaking toward the bull's rump. I'm wishing it along, not daring to hope it will actually reach the animal.

"*Tsaa,* got it!" I call. The dart is firmly stuck in the rump muscles. The tension in my body eases, my hand relaxes, and I draw a deep, grateful breath. "Take it easy. Slow down and let him get some space, no need to scare him any further."

Slowly the intense cold is returning and my nose is now perfectly numb. *Got to watch out for frostbite,* I think. But no matter, we have our first camel.

In the distance, the bull nearly vanishes from sight in the driving snow. Then he slows and assumes a drunken pacing. He's fighting the drug effects, but I know we have him this time. After a few more minutes, he sinks to the ground and lies down. We wait, letting the drugs take their full effect.

"Looks good. His breathing is regular and deep," Petra says as she fixes the bull with her binoculars. I get out of the jeep, shoulder the medical pack, and walk across the snow-driven plain. My patient is rapidly disappearing in a snowdrift. He does not react to gentle prodding; I wave to the others to join me.

I get down on my knees and look the bull in the open eyes while I place my pulse oximeter probe on his tongue. Beep, beep, beep, the reassuring heartbeats resound above the wind. He's at 94 percent saturation, which is near normal for the oxygen levels in his blood, despite the anesthesia. I stroke the bull's tousled hairy head and say quietly, "It's going to be all right."

Petra is kneeling next to me in the snow. Though she has her face mask on, I can see in her eyes that she is smiling. "Okay?" she asks.

"Yeah, start putting on the collar. I'll try to get a blood sample." I search with my finger for the jugular vein. "What a hairy beast," I mutter. "This blood sample is not going to be simple." Finally, the needle slips into the vein; the first few drops of blood appear and then instantly freeze. "Petra, this is not going to work—the blood is freezing in the needle."

"Hang on, I have some warm needles in my fleece." She hands me one.

It works. The blood slowly fills the tube, and we have our first good genetic sample. The Global Positioning System (GPS) unit mounted on top of the collar will determine the bull's location three times a day and transmit the data to our field station every other day via the French Argos satellite system. With this information, we will be able to learn more about the bull's movement patterns and determine his requirements for space and food. This data is essential if we have any hope of conserving this species for future generations. Mounted on the side of the collar is an additional unit, a small explosive charge that will activate sixteen months from now to release the collar. This sounds dangerous to the animal, but the very small charge is carefully contained in a steel casing that channels the explosion to simply remove a retaining pin. Similar collars have been used in all kinds of smaller, more fragile species like elk and deer.

The bull's head seems to be floating above the snow. The rest of his scruffy, dark brown body is covered by the snowdrift.

"We're all done," I announce. "Let's get this animal up before he's completely snowed in." One by one, my team members approach the bull, stroking his head. Each bids the camel good-bye in his or her own way, wishing him well for his future travels in the Gobi.

I am alone with the bull, holding the syringe filled with the reversal drug. Once it's in the vein, the animal will awaken and shortly thereafter jump up—and most probably run off. The needle once again slips into the vein and I depress the plunger. My knee is firmly on the bull's lower jaw, fixing his head to the ground. I don't want him attempting to get up before he has the strength to throw me off.

The bull and I have been together for the past hour. The chase, the dart, and the hairy head in the snow are etched in my mind. Once he leaves to roam the Gobi, I hope that he will never again meet another human.

He begins to stir, his breaths deepen, and then he makes a first feeble attempt to throw me off. "You will have to do better than that," I say. Finally, a few minutes later, the bull wheezes noisily and throws me into the snow. He looks slightly confused, but holds his head high and glares at me. This typical camel look lets me know he is back in charge. He gets up and takes a few wide-legged, shaky steps away from me before stopping and turning back one last time.

"Go on, be well and take care," I tell him. "We will be watching you."

The bull turns away, disappearing again into the driving snow.

Six months later, in the comfort of my Vienna office, I log on to the Argos satellite Web page to check up on the collared bull. It's summer in the Gobi, where daytime temperatures often reach 50° centigrade (122° Fahrenheit). The camel is moving north, tracking rainfall and good pasture. Remarkably, we've yet to see any signs of illness or injury in this bull or in any of the other five collared animals, despite the harsh conditions in the desert. Though our data is preliminary, one thing is clear: this remarkable species needs a great deal of space in order to remain healthy and survive.

ABOUT THE AUTHOR

Christian Walzer has been a professor at the Research Institute of Wildlife Ecology, University of Veterinary Medicine, in Austria, since 2005. He earned his veterinary degree from the University of Veterinary Medicine, Vienna, in 1990. Since that time, he has worked in rural practice and served as the zoological codirector, head veterinarian, and staff researcher at Zoo Salzburg in Austria. Dr. Walzer is recognized internationally for his expertise in working with wildlife, especially wild equids and carnivores, gained from combined years of work and study in Europe, Asia, and Africa. He has participated in numerous challenging field projects, including the transporting of Przewalski's horses from Europe to Mongolia, the study of the impact of human intrusion on the khulan (wild ass) in the Gobi Desert, and the placement of satellite-monitoring collars on wild camels. He is currently conducting various research projects in Mongolia, including landscape-level research for the conservation of the Asiatic wild ass, funded by the Austrian Science Foundation.

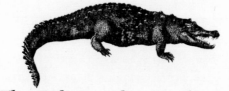

The Bikers, the Students, and the Crocodile

by Juergen Schumacher, DVM

Becoming a crocodile veterinarian was not on my priority list when I attended veterinary school in Germany. I'd always wanted to become a zoo vet, but working with reptiles, particularly snakes and crocodiles, wasn't what I'd ever envisioned. Though I'd grown up with many animals, including dogs, hamsters, birds, fish, and a tortoise, my mother might have given me away for adoption had I come home with a snake!

But everything changed when reptiles first became my patients. They are fascinating creatures, and as I began to appreciate their place in the animal kingdom, I acquired my own reptiles, especially tortoises. To this day, they are my passion.

I'm lucky that my wife shares my fascination with reptiles and has allowed me to keep quite a few of them. However, there is one major problem associated with my reptile keeping: many species, especially the tortoise, are very long lived. Sometime in the future I will have to make the necessary arrangements to put them in my will.

The veterinary hospital where I worked during the mid-1990s provided medical care to exotic animals kept as pets, including birds, reptiles, and small mammals, as well as wildlife patients. We also provided care for several zoological parks. One of these institutions, the St. Augustine Alligator Farm Zoological Park in St. Augustine, Florida, had a two-thousand-pound male saltwater crocodile named Gomek in its collection. He was approximately 17.5 feet in length, with a V-shaped head the size of my dinner table. Dark scales covered most of his body and huge, peglike teeth lined his jaws.

Considering his enormous size (saltwater crocodiles are the world's largest reptile), Gomek was surprisingly docile. He performed daily for tourists from all over the world during his scheduled feeding sessions. It was an amazing spectacle, actually, to watch an animal of his size gently take food items from the end of a long hook held by a zookeeper—not at all what you'd expect after watching some of the nature shows about wild crocodiles.

On my regular visits to the zoo, I'd often pass by the crocodile exhibit. Gomek appeared to be in good health, so there was little work for me to do. Sometimes we'd review his husbandry—routine feeding, cleaning, and housing protocols—with the zookeepers and curator. The crocodile was fed a variety of food items; he especially liked nutria, a member of the rodent family. He lived by himself in a large enclosure with a spacious pool where visitors could observe him through an underwater viewing area.

On one such visit, the curator asked me to take a closer look at what appeared to be a skin infection on Gomek's tail. From a safe distance, I could see patchy white areas along the edges, or margins, of several scales near the base of his tail. The lesions looked superficial, but we agreed to keep a close eye on the condition. I suspected some type of bacterial or fungal infection and hoped it would resolve on its own, but it didn't. Though the skin problem didn't seem to bother the crocodile, the number of affected scales increased over the next few months. We decided to treat him empirically (based on observation) with antibiotics rather than put him—and us—through the stress of an exam.

Selecting an effective antibiotic for a reptile is often a challenge because little information is available on which drug is most effective and how frequently it should be given. Also, different reptile species vary tremendously in weight, ranging from a few grams (e.g., a gecko) to one ton (e.g., a saltwater crocodile). Thus the amount of antibiotic and the route of delivery vary depending on the patient.

Our initial thought was to hide the antibiotic in the crocodile's food. But we knew this form of administration might not be very effective in this species. A large cold-blooded reptile has a lower body temperature and thus a lower metabolic rate than a similarly sized warm-blooded mammal. These physiologic differences mean that reptiles metabolize drugs more slowly and/or less completely. Most antibiotics given orally to crocodiles are not well absorbed and may not reach therapeutic levels. The head reptile keeper felt

comfortable giving the crocodile intramuscular injections using a syringe attached to an eight-foot pole, though. This route
of antibiotic therapy is often effective in treating bacterial skin
diseases in reptiles. So we planned to try it for a month.

After about four weeks of treatment, I called the zoo as
usual the day before my regularly scheduled visit and spoke
with the head reptile keeper. We discussed the crocodile's
skin condition, which hadn't improved despite the antibiotics. The good news was that Gomek was active and certainly hadn't lost his appetite. The major shortcoming of our
treatment regimen was that we'd tried treating the problem
without a definite diagnosis. So I suggested to the head
keeper that we anesthetize the crocodile sometime soon to
collect appropriate diagnostic samples. We needed to determine whether the lesions were bacterial and/or fungal in ori-
gin. From there, we could initiate more specific therapy.
Despite the potential risks of anesthesia, he agreed. We
planned to have me look at the animal again and then arrange
for a full workup in the near future.

Anesthesia in large reptiles poses a number of challenges,
however. Crocodiles and alligators command the same respect as lions and tigers when it comes to working with them
in close quarters—all are potentially dangerous carnivores.
Despite the differences in metabolic rate between reptiles
and mammals, some anesthetics work reasonably well in both
classes of animal. Other anesthetic drugs may have very little
effect, while some, if not dosed precisely, can inadvertently
kill the patient.

Once anesthetized, reptiles also behave differently from
mammals. Their heart and breathing rates during anesthesia

tend to be extremely low, making it hard to judge anesthetic depth. Gomek, for example, might breathe only once every few minutes during anesthesia, and his heart rate might decrease below two beats per minute. If we did decide to anesthetize him, we'd need to be extremely careful for his safety—and mine.

The next morning, I left the hospital with a group of senior veterinary students who were looking forward to a field trip that would get them out of the clinic. They also seemed enthusiastic about the prospect of a nice lunch at the beach after we finished work at the zoo. We arrived early and completed most of our scheduled rounds by late morning, including rechecks of other patients that were being treated for a variety of conditions. Then it was time to check the crocodile.

I gathered the students and we headed down the walkway to Gomek's enclosure. At that time my plan was just to have another look at him and talk to the staff about when and how to anesthetize the crocodile for further diagnostics. On my way to the enclosure, I noticed a large number of leather-clad bikers on the zoo grounds. I was informed by the zoo staff that there was an annual biker meeting in a town nearby and that many had received free passes to the zoo. As a result, there seemed to be more bikers than animals on the grounds.

When we approached the crocodile's enclosure, I was surprised to see that the pool had been drained and that the huge reptile was resting motionless at the bottom. Not immediately realizing what was going on, I looked at the head keeper questioningly. He explained that he'd drained it overnight so that he and I could simply climb down to the bottom of the pool. There I could examine the crocodile and collect my diagnostic samples.

I tried to erase from my memory all the images I'd seen on various documentaries that demonstrated what crocodiles are capable of doing to their prey. Fortunately, the *Crocodile Hunter* show hadn't started on television yet; otherwise, my plan of action might have been very different. Sensing that I was a little nervous about the situation, the head keeper quickly told me that the procedure would be perfectly safe. Meanwhile the students were listening and watching in disbelief that I was even considering climbing down into a pool to examine this giant animal. I must have been thinking, in the back of my mind, that the risks of anesthetizing this tremendously popular crocodile outweighed the benefits—and I also trusted the keeper.

I decided to do the examination; I also decided that if I felt unsafe at any point, I would abort the procedure. I left the students outside the enclosure and instructed them just to watch (hoping they wouldn't have an exciting story to tell their friends and family about a stupid veterinarian they once knew . . .). I collected my instruments, including forceps, scissors, scalpel blade, biopsy needle, and sample collection tubes, and followed on the heels of the unconcerned keeper. When we arrived at the bottom of the pool, about ten feet below ground level and only a few feet away from Gomek, the crocodile appeared even larger than he did through the viewing window.

Though I hadn't paid too much attention to the bikers, I noticed now that a large group was watching the three of us—me, the crocodile, and the keeper—through the underwater viewing window. From their curious expressions, I knew they must have been wondering what was going on: What in the world was I intending to do with this crocodile?

I quickly returned my attention to the animal, which still hadn't moved and appeared to be oblivious to our presence. As a precaution, I considered my escape strategy while I was still relatively calm and collected, which is always a good idea, since the human brain has a tendency not to work very well in moments of panic. I would be at the base of the crocodile's tail while I took my samples. His head was in the corner; if he spun around to get me, I figured he would hit the viewing glass first. This would, I hoped, buy me the split second I'd need to jump away from him and climb back out of the enclosure. In retrospect, it wasn't a very intelligent plan. One whip of his large, powerful tail probably would have broken several of my bones and sent me flying out of the enclosure.

Using the forceps and blade, I was able to remove several full-thickness biopsy specimens of the diseased scales for later examination under a microscope (histopathology). I also scraped the surface of Gomek's skin for bacterial and fungal cultures. My patient barely moved during the procedure. But I began to feel nervous toward the end. After looking into the crocodile's dark yellow eyes, I realized that I really do not like being part of the food chain.

Finishing my sample collection, I quickly climbed out of the enclosure and began to place the tissue samples and swabs in vials. The keeper followed up after me. Looking over my shoulder, down the side of the pool, and into the crocodile's emotionless eyes, then back at my samples, I suddenly realized what I'd just done, and my hands began to shake. Somehow, I managed to place my samples into the tubes without dropping them.

As we left the enclosure, the students looked at me wide-eyed, without saying a word. The group of bikers who had watched the whole procedure through the glass quickly approached us. They were all dressed in jeans, boots, and leather jackets; most of the guys had full beards. They looked at us silently for several seconds, studying our faces. It was obvious that they had plenty of questions but couldn't decide who would actually do the talking. Finally, one of them asked, "Is he dead?"

I shook my head. "He is alive and fine."

The bikers stared at me in disbelief. "What did you give him?" the same guy asked. "He's asleep, right?"

"No, I didn't give the crocodile anything. He is absolutely awake."

The group looked at each other, obviously thinking the same thing. The spokesman glared at me, shook his head, and said, "You are stupid, boy. You are really stupid." The rest of the group nodded in support, then walked away, undoubtedly agreeing that all veterinarians with foreign accents are stupid.

As I packed up my equipment, I realized that my students also were staring at me. They must have been wondering why I was still alive, if this was how I worked with dangerous animals. A bit embarrassed, and not entirely sure how to explain the whole episode to them, I calmly told them that what they had just witnessed was not something they should try if they wanted to reach regular retirement age. I also added that it wasn't something I planned to do ever again without proper restraint of the animal.

We had one more group of animals to examine before we were done for the day, a bale of tortoises. When we arrived at their enclosure, these harmless reptiles were obviously happy to greet this large group of visitors. The whole group walked up to us, looking for food, investigating our shoes and bags, and presenting their necks so we could scratch them. We all relaxed during our visit with these friendly animals (particularly me!), and I'm sure the tortoises enjoyed the attention.

In retrospect, though, the crocodile had proved to be an equally cooperative patient. And his skin lesions did eventually heal. We grew several organisms from the samples, including a bacteria that was resistant to our earlier choice of antibiotics. We changed his medicine to one that would target this specific bacteria and, based on recent studies in other reptiles, would work orally. Gomek readily took the antibiotics in his food. Within a few weeks, the lesions began to resolve.

My decision to climb into a dry pool to examine a fully awake giant crocodile occurred at the beginning of my career. It remains a vivid memory; even years later, I often tell this story to friends and colleagues. Now, after working with a variety of potentially dangerous animals over the years, I would not go into the pool under similar circumstances. This case taught me to assess each animal and situation differently. At the time, I didn't have the experience or maturity to say no to the procedure, though I never felt completely safe. Eventually, I learned to think about my well-being—and sometimes not to listen to other people. I still plan to put my tortoises in my will.

ABOUT THE AUTHOR

Juergen Schumacher was born in Germany and graduated from the College of Veterinary Medicine, University of Berlin, in 1988. The following year, he moved to the United States for his graduate studies at the College of Veterinary Medicine, University of Florida, where he completed residencies in both anesthesiology and zoological medicine. In 1997, he joined the faculty at the College of Veterinary Medicine, University of Tennessee, and is currently an associate professor and service chief of the Avian and Zoological Medicine Service. He teaches zoo-animal medicine and has published dozens of scientific articles and book chapters on various topics in zoological medicine. Dr. Schumacher is board certified by the American College of Zoological Medicine and holds German board certification in reptile medicine and surgery. His clinical and research interests are anesthesia and analgesia of zoo animals as well as reptile medicine and surgery. Though he enjoys working with all species, tortoises are by far his favorite.

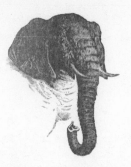

Tracking a Snared Elephant

by Sharon Deem, DVM, PhD

Veterinarians face the same questions every day: What is wrong with this animal? How will I solve its problem? Should I treat it, and if so, when? How can I prevent the problem from happening again? This is true of our job whether we take care of dogs and cats or hermit crabs and elephants. Our patients don't tell us what they need or where they hurt, and we can't tell them that we're there to help. Often, just getting started is half the battle. In my experience, a dart gun loaded with anesthetic is the only way to convince an injured wild elephant, for example, that it needs to see a doctor.

When I took the call from the woman in a nearby town, I knew we were in for a challenge. She described a free-ranging bull forest elephant with a snare wrapped around his lower left leg. At the time, in 2005, my husband, my son, and

I were living in Libreville, in the central African country of Gabon. I was working as a research veterinarian for the Smithsonian's National Zoo. My husband, Steve, was a field biologist for the Wildlife Conservation Society. Our two-year-old son, Charlie, was busy growing up in one of the most beautiful countries on earth, learning English and French with youthful enthusiasm and ease.

Together, Steve and I had studied the behavior and movements of healthy forest elephants, anesthetizing several of them for the placement of GPS tracking collars—work that was part of a larger ecological study led by Steve to gather much-needed data on forest elephant home ranges and habitat use. We had not, however, treated an injured free-ranging elephant within the forest. This was a whole new ball game.

The woman asked, "Would it be possible to remove the snare before the elephant becomes aggressive to people—or before someone in the village kills him because he is an easy target?"

The African forest elephant, *Loxodonta africana cyclotis*, lives only in the rain forest of central and west Africa. Threatened by poaching for ivory and meat and by habitat fragmentation due to logging and mining, this subspecies of elephant faces an uncertain future. Here in the dense jungle of Gabon, snare hunting is an all-too-frequent method of capturing a number of wildlife species. The indiscriminate snare often results in a slow, painful, and horrific death.

Steve and I discussed the situation. We were willing to give it a try. Our major concern was that we lacked an essential tool: a team of trackers. Our philosophy had always been that if you can't find your elephant after you have anesthetized it, you shouldn't anesthetize it in the first place! The Pygmy people of central Africa have exceptional tracking skills. During our earlier elephant work, we'd been assisted by a team of BaAka Pygmies, but there was no way to reassemble them quickly enough for this patient. Fortunately, we found two Gabonese guards working for the World Wildlife Fund who agreed to help with tracking. Without them, I doubt we would even have tried to dart the elephant.

We flew to the coastal town of Gamba, set up our gear at the building that would serve as our home and laboratory, and met with local people to hear what they knew about the lame elephant's condition and current whereabouts. In late afternoon, the team started its search; several hours after sunset, we caught our first glimpse of the injured elephant, limping across the savanna about thirty feet from where we stood. Using our flashlights, we could see he was a beautiful adult bull elephant in the prime of life (we estimated him to be in his midtwenties), standing approximately eight feet at the shoulders with short, straight tusks. More important, we could see a band of constricted skin and muscle around his lower left front leg.

I knew instantly that we didn't have much time before the animal would develop a bone infection, osteomyelitis, or irreversible tissue damage to the foot from lack of blood flow. At that point, treatment would be futile. As soon as possible, I had to get in a position where I could safely dart this elephant.

We spent our second day searching for him. As night fell, he reappeared, walking out from the forest into the savanna. He was almost within range, in a clear area, and my dart gun was loaded. All I had to do was get a bit closer. I felt incredibly lucky. Just twenty-four hours after the search began, we'd soon have our patient on the "operating ground," anesthetized for snare removal and wound treatment. Or so I thought.

Unfortunately, the elephant saw us and limped away as quickly as his painful leg would allow. The remaining daylight was fading fast. Though I knew my position now was less than ideal, I fired—and missed. At that point, I had no choice but to accept the fact that evening conditions were not safe for either people or elephants. I elected not to shoot again. It was a blow to our team. No one spoke as we walked back to the truck; I wondered if the others were thinking, *How could she miss a target the size of an elephant?*

During the next four days, we covered a great deal of ground on foot and by truck, hoping to find the elephant again so I could safely dart him, ideally in a clearing away from water during daylight hours. We followed tracks and various leads given to us from people living in the area. We looked specifically for signs of our lame bull. From the size and spacing of the footprints, we could differentiate a forest elephant with a normal gait from one with a limp.

On several occasions, we sat for hours near patches of forest where we had calculated that the elephant had entered, or where we thought he would exit. Despite our efforts, we could not find him. Maybe he wouldn't give us that second chance. Frustrated, tired, and worried, we knew we were running out of time. We had lost our elephant.

On the evening of the fifth day, the elephant found us. Limping badly, he walked out of the forest and through a clearing about one hundred feet from our truck, just as the team was preparing to end the day's search. I had been standing, ready and waiting with my dart gun, near this spot for hours prior to the elephant's bold move. As he walked past me in the fading light, we all knew there was no chance of safely darting him. Thirty seconds later, he had entered the forest on the far side of the clearing and again disappeared from sight. I disassembled my gun and packed up my equipment; this was the end of yet another frustrating day. Could the elephant be smarter than our entire team?

The elephant must have been waiting among the dense trees, watching us. Maybe he chose that particular time to cross the clearing because he knew that as darkness fell, I would not again attempt to dart him. Maybe he knew that we could no longer follow his tracks for the rest of the night. Did he also know that my gun and anesthetic drug were part of a plan to help, rather than cause him harm? I wanted to believe that this animal understood—on some level—what we were trying to do for him. Maybe he'd come out from the forest to let us know he was still alive. Or maybe he was simply ready to walk from one side of the clearing to the other, and our presence had nothing to do with it. We resumed our search the next morning.

Two days later, we closed in on our patient once again. His movements had slowed, and he now spent most of his time in, or near, a small lake. I sat for hours on the water's edge watching him from a distance. He would swim into the center, presumably to take weight off the painful leg. Then he would return to the shore, fill his trunk with lake water, and squirt it over the wound, cleaning it—his own method of administering hydrotherapy. He repeated this treatment many times throughout the day. I watched in amazement and admiration. The elephant showed me something we very rarely observe: self-treatment by an animal patient. Sadly, he couldn't remove the metal snare on his own. It was also obvious that his lameness had worsened and that the swelling had increased significantly in the area around the snare. I was determined to help him, no matter what it took.

We could no longer wait for the perfect opportunity; there might never be one. After much discussion, Steve and I decided that darting the animal on the lake's edge was our only option. Our biggest concern was that, once darted, the elephant would immediately rush into the center of the lake. If this happened, we would have to somehow force him to change course before the anesthesia took effect. Otherwise, he would surely drown. We would need to devise a plan.

The following day, with Steve and one of the trackers, I moved into a patch of forest on the lake's edge. There we sat and waited, watching the elephant resting in the lake as he had the day before. After several hours, he moved to the bank and began to feed on the vegetation within reach of his trunk. We knew this was our best chance. I would have to take this shot if we were to have any chance of saving our patient's life.

Slowly advancing along the edge of the lake, using the trees for cover, I cut the distance down to about 175 feet. Not ideal—half that distance would have been better—but good enough, I hoped. The elephant looked in my direction; he sensed my presence and seemed almost as nervous as I felt. It was time to pull the trigger. I fired and the dart hit him in the middle of the left thigh muscle. From where I stood, it appeared that the anesthetic had been injected. A perfect shot!

Now my mind was racing. We had to track him from a safe distance, but close enough to ensure we could reach the elephant soon after the drug took effect. Most important, we needed to keep him out of the deep water. The elephant ran straight toward the center of the lake, just as we'd anticipated. But Steve had devised an ingenious plan the night before. He radioed the second tracker, who was waiting in a small motorboat around the bend in the lake. As the boat sped out into the open lake, the elephant changed his course and swam away from the boat, toward the forest edge.

We struggled to keep up with him, running in hip-deep water, our adrenaline pumping. When he disappeared into the trees, we raced after his footprints. The next forty-five minutes felt like hours and seconds all in one. Without Pygmy trackers, Steve and I had worried that our own tracking skills would not be sufficient to lead us to the elephant. We ran through the thick forest unable to see our patient, sweat blurring our vision, branches cutting our faces and limbs. It was only from the sounds of breaking trees and rustling bushes ahead that we knew he was not yet anesthetized.

Most forest elephants we've darted go down under the effects of the drug within twenty minutes. Thirty minutes into the chase, I decided to make a second dart, concerned that the first one might not have injected the drug properly and that we were in fact chasing a fully awake, injured elephant. Standing in a small clearing as I prepared my equipment, I could hear him moving just inside the forest cover. Then there was no sound. Had he moved on? Was he standing there by the forest edge waiting for us to come in after him? Was he okay? Why hadn't they taught me this in vet school?

When the second dart was ready, we all headed back into the trees. The elephant had disappeared once again. We raced after his footprints. Forty minutes after I'd fired the first dart back at the lake, we heard heavy breathing and the rustling sounds of branches just a few feet ahead of us. Then we spotted the elephant lying down but attempting to stand. It appeared that the anesthesia I'd used was not a high enough dose. The elephant was fighting the effects of the morphine-like drug. Severe pain combined with high levels of stress can override this anesthetic. His adrenaline levels—like ours—must have been off the charts by this time.

Cautiously, I approached the elephant from the rear and hand-injected a second dose of anesthetic. Two minutes later, our patient was finally ready for treatment.

We removed the snare, cleaned the wound, applied topical antibiotic, administered a tetanus vaccine, and gave him an elephant-sized injection of long-acting antibiotic. His foot appeared viable: the tissues bled easily and there was no bone exposed—both excellent signs. I also collected a blood sample that we later analyzed to assess his general health. Once the team was a safe distance away, I gave the elephant his anesthetic reversal.

Three minutes later, he was standing and walking away from us. For the first time, he was doing exactly what we wanted him to do.

Had my patient been in a zoo, I would have scheduled

twice-daily treatments and daily antibiotic injections. But of course, elephants don't run into poaching snares in zoos, nor do they require their doctors to track them for eight days in the jungle. Here we could only rely on a onetime dose of medicine, the elephant's self-treatments, and time. With the snare off, at least he had a chance. I'm thankful that my veterinary skills could help save at least one animal from this terrible and cruel fate.

The elephant, whom I'd named Tobbie Deux after my twenty-one-year-old three-legged cat, was seen later the same day of treatment as well as many times since. He no longer has a limp, but the scar remains, a reminder to him—and to us—of the snare that could have killed him. When he looks at the scar, I wonder if it reminds him of the humans who set the snare, or the four-person team who chased him for eight days and saved his life. I'd like to believe it's the latter.

ABOUT THE AUTHOR

Sharon L. Deem has conducted conservation and research projects for captive and free-ranging wildlife in nineteen countries around the world. Dr. Deem received her bachelor's degree in biology from Virginia Polytechnic Institute and State University, her doctorate in veterinary medicine from Virginia–Maryland Regional College of Veterinary Medicine, and her PhD in veterinary epidemiology from the University of Florida, where she also completed a three-year zoo and wildlife medicine residency. Dr. Deem is board certified by the American College of Zoological Medicine.

Her interests in wildlife veterinary medicine focus on the spread of disease between domestic animals and wildlife and the impact of environmental changes and human contact on the health and conservation of wild species. She is the author of over fifty journal articles, ten book chapters, and numerous other papers. Dr. Deem currently works for the St. Louis Zoo's WildCare Institute as a veterinary epidemiologist. She; her husband, Dr. Stephen Blake; and their son, Charlie, recently moved to the Galápagos Islands for their next adventure.

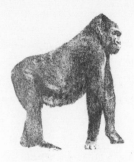

Partners in the Mist: A Close Call

by Christopher Whittier, DVM,

with Felicia Nutter, DVM, PhD

Few people are fortunate enough to realize their dream jobs. Even fewer are able to do so in partnership with their spouses. When Felicia and I were given that opportunity as field veterinarians for the Mountain Gorilla Veterinary Project (MGVP), we knew there was more than enough work for us both, but we weren't sure exactly how we would divide it.

Our second case in the field, just three weeks after Felicia joined me in Rwanda in December 2002, proved a major test of our teamwork. It involved a young adult male gorilla that had recently been forced out of his group. Ironically, he was named Joliami, the French translation of "nice friend," something he turned out not to be.

There are no books on gorilla medicine. Because they are

so similar to humans, and such valuable members of any cap-tive collection, most zoo gorillas receive cutting-edge treat-ment from highly specialized human and veterinary medical experts. In the wild, gorilla medicine is more like giving first aid on a battlefield, usually in the rain.

The mandate of MGVP is to intervene with wild gorillas only when cases are life threatening or human-induced. The biggest threats to their health include injuries to hands or feet from poachers' snares and exposure to human infectious diseases, particularly flulike respiratory disease, introduced by park visitors. But sometimes even minor injuries can de-velop into serious conditions. This leaves a fair amount of ambiguity and interpretation in deciding whether to treat the animal or not, a situation that can be both good and bad from the field veterinarian's perspective.

In this case, Joliami had suffered many severe cuts and lac-erations all over his body. The cause of his injuries was un-known, but they were most likely the result of a fight with one or more gorillas, a circumstance that normally does not warrant intervention. There was a remote possibility that he had been caught in a vicious type of poachers' trap used to maim and capture wild buffalo, but this scenario seemed less likely.

We discussed the situation with the park staff, the govern-ment officials who oversee the Parc National des Volcans in Rwanda, and other conservation partners. Ultimately the de-cision to intervene was based on the fact that Joliami had such severe wounds on both hands that he was unable to walk or to eat properly. We feared he could lose multiple fingers, perhaps even most of his hands, which would doom him to starvation and death. Additionally, the population had recently suffered the poaching deaths of almost a dozen healthy gorillas. The stakeholders felt that saving one young silverback (adult male gorilla), even if endangered only by natural injuries, would be worthwhile.

Felicia made the initial solo check after the report of Joliami's injuries. He was in such a miserable state that she immediately administered antibiotic treatment with darts. On her return, she raised the possibility of intervening surgically to deal with his wounds. We discussed the issue and decided to mobilize a full intervention team for the following day, which happened to be New Year's Eve.

We gathered our backpacks full of medical equipment and started early in the morning, with the famous Virunga Volcanoes still draped in mist. The team included the two of us, along with the Rwandan park's veterinary technician, Elisabeth Nyirakaragire; an Australian behavioral research intern, Graham Wallace; and several of the most experienced of the gorilla park staff, including the highly respected Faustin Barabwiriza from the Karisoke Research Center.

Barabwiriza had been hired by Dian Fossey as a young camp assistant before rising through the ranks to become the leader of the team that followed Joliami's group. He was invaluable for his familiarity with the individual gorillas, including Joliami, but not easy for us to communicate with because he knew no English and only a little French. It had been years since Felicia or I had studied Swahili, and we struggled to learn Kinyarwanda. Still, we could usually muster enough common language to communicate during our field days with Barabwiriza, if only because when at work he was a man of few words. Much of his communication was via nods and gestures, and sometimes a disappointed shake of his head when we misidentified an individual gorilla that was as familiar to him as a member of his own family. At parties, after downing a giant Primus beer, a different Barabwiriza emerged, this one often first onto the dance floor, a huge grin on his face as he performed one of the traditional Rwandan men's dances, stomping along to the drums in his knee-high rubber boots. This dichotomy, along with his history and experience, had already endeared him to us.

Although we were hiking up to Joliami's vicinity fully prepared for immobilization and treatment, we needed to reassess his condition first before making a final decision to intervene. One of the nice aspects of working as a team was that Felicia and I could discuss such cases and make our decisions together. In this instance, she elected not to influence my impressions of Joliami's condition, saying I should have a first look at him with Graham and Barabwiriza before comparing notes with what she'd seen the previous day.

The three of us found the injured gorilla about twenty meters off the trail, sitting with his hands tucked into his chest and licking his wounds. I knew Joliami from previous years but had not seen him for a while. Like most male gorillas approaching adulthood, he'd been something of a prankster, liking to show off his bravery and strength by toying with human visitors—pushing them around, trying to remove their backpacks. Of course, this degree of contact is discouraged for both human and gorilla safety, but it's not always easy to follow the rules in the home of a three-hundred-pound gorilla intent on doing as he pleases. Though these encounters could sometimes be dangerous, it was hard to take Joliami very seriously, in part because he had oversized, prominent ears that gave him a cartoonish, goofy look.

But he was no joke on this visit. The previous day, he'd been so miserable that he'd sat and let Felicia shoot two darts into him without resistance. He'd simply groaned as the first dart hit his right thigh, then feebly moved about six feet away. At the sound of the soft *pifft* made by the CO_2 gun as it fired again, he'd turned his head to follow the flight of the second dart as it landed in his left thigh. Usually the injection of ten milliliters of thick penicillin from each dart stung enough to elicit a response from the patient, but Joliami remained listless.

Today when we approached, he immediately grunted a loud warning vocalization, then showed us he didn't want company by grabbing on to a small tree and snapping it down onto Barabwiriza's head. This is typical behavior for a silverback. Barabwiriza responded to this threat with a grin at the impertinence of this gorilla he'd known since birth.

Though Joliami had regained some of his usual energy overnight, probably the result of the antibiotics beginning to work, his condition was still very serious. After a brief discussion we decided to go ahead with the planned intervention. Moving up a trail out of the gorilla's line of sight, Felicia and I prepared the darts and reminded the team of everyone's role and responsibility. Felicia was always good about letting me play gun-toter, and this day was no different, especially since she'd had the opportunity the day before— Joliami presumably had little interest in seeing her again.

In theory, this intervention would be easier than most

because there were no other gorillas around to interfere with our work. But we were also immobilizing a full-sized and, at the moment, quite ornery silverback, a procedure that would require two carefully placed anesthetic darts. I tried to lighten the tension by joking about Barabwiriza's stoic reputation, saying, "If you hear anyone scream, it's Barabwiriza." Unfortunately, the joke turned into reality in only a few minutes, though others would do the screaming.

Returning to where we'd left Joliami, we got a quick opportunity and delivered the first dart into his shoulder. To our surprise, he immediately rose and departed, moving much more quickly than we'd thought he could. We followed him as he climbed onto the trail above, uphill from where we'd left the rest of the team. One of the first rules of gorilla darting is never to dart *any* gorilla when there is a silverback uphill of you, let alone a silverback himself. Another obvious rule is to hide your equipment. No animal wants to see the barrel of gun pointing in its direction, and few ever forget. The previous day, with Joliami depressed and lethargic, Felicia had been able to violate both rules with impunity.

As Joliami moved up the trail, he gave me a perfect rear leg target. Impelled by the urgency of landing that second dart, I made the regrettable decision to shoot from what I knew was a vulnerable position. I waited until he turned and headed uphill, but just as I was raising the dart gun, he glanced back and saw it pointed at him. He immediately charged down the trail, screaming.

We are taught to hold our ground on a charging gorilla, but that really only applies to bluff charges—which this was not. We had a mere second to react. My own best chance was

to make a bullfighter's move and dodge him at the last second, hoping his momentum would propel him down the trail
into a less dangerous position. This worked for me, and, on
the opposite side of the trail, for Barabwiriza. Unlucky
Graham had nowhere to go, with the two of us occupying the
only openings in the thick brush. Joliami wrapped his arms
around Graham's legs and tackled him to the ground.

Joliami's and then Graham's screams sent most of the intervention team into rapid flight. Only Felicia and Elisabeth
held their positions. From about thirty meters downhill and
around a curve, they couldn't see what was happening, but
they knew from the sound that someone was being savaged.
Quickly they grabbed the heavy bags full of drugs and medical equipment and ran up the trail to help, wondering which
one of us they'd find at the business end of the angry gorilla.

I sat frozen for those few seconds, helplessly watching
Graham in Joliami's clutches, envisioning Robert Shaw's
character sliding into the mouth of the shark in *Jaws* and
thinking I would be next. Barabwiriza, on the other hand,
fully lived up to his reputation. He ran across the trail and repeatedly booted Joliami in the rear end as hard as he could
until the gorilla moved. Seemingly stunned by this affront,
possibly recognizing that Barabwiriza outranked him, and
with the partial dose of anesthetic starting to work, Joliami
released his hold on Graham, stepped over him, and tumbled
into a dry streambed a few steps away.

Another advantage of working together as a team is the
ability to divide and conquer, which fortuitously came into
play here. Graham, starting to go into shock, was helped
to his feet and said he thought he'd been bitten. Though his

rain-pants were not torn, a quick examination underneath them revealed that one of Joliami's huge canine teeth had caused a single deep puncture in the fold of Graham's thigh near the large artery and veins that supply the leg, severely bruising the surrounding muscles but, fortunately, not damaging any vital structures. He needed immediate medical care as well as quick arrangements to get him the couple thousand feet down the side of the mountain before his adrenaline ran out and he began to feel even more pain. But we also had a partially anesthetized gorilla that required treatment. With little need for discussion, Felicia attended to Graham while Barabwiriza and I went after Joliami and got the rest of his anesthetic dose into him.

Before long, Graham was hobbling down the trail to meet a rescue vehicle with the support of several strong porters, Joliami was in the streambed with the second dart taking effect, and the whole team—minus Graham—was reunited for the job we'd come to do.

As the more thorough, careful, observant, and detail-oriented member of our partnership, Felicia took control of Joliami's anesthesia as planned. She placed a breathing tube into his trachea in order to ensure steady breathing and also to enable us to use gas anesthesia, something that had not been traditionally done with wild mountain gorillas. With assistance from Elisabeth, she continually monitored his breathing and heart rate, occasionally supplementing the anesthetic from the darts with isoflurane gas through our improvised field delivery system.

As the arguably more dexterous partner with slightly more hands-on surgery experience, I performed the bulk of the wound repairs, trying to close Joliami's major cuts after a thorough cleaning and debriding of dead and infected tissues. Murphy's Law dictated the onset of rain just as this was under way, so part of the surgery was performed under an improvised tarpaulin rain-cover. I decided to partially close the deep lacerations on Joliami's forearm and both hands with sutures, leaving openings for drainage to help prevent abscessation but also because some areas were simply too swollen. We were relieved to find no damage to the tendons that open and close a gorilla's immensely powerful hands and fingers, nor were any bones or joints exposed. This was good news for Joliami's prognosis.

While I was suturing, Felicia prepped the next wound; while I was drawing blood for samples, she administered additional antibiotic doses. Close communication and a reliable support team made for a smooth and successful field procedure, despite all that had previously occurred.

We waited as long as possible for Joliami to start waking from the anesthetic, but knew we couldn't take many more chances with such a formidable patient. Felicia removed his breathing tube and we tried to set him in a safe position. We left him covered with the tarp in view of the increasing rain and his lowered body temperature from the anesthesia. Though we'd been working in cramped quarters in the deep, narrow ravine, the location was beneficial for the gorilla's recovery, as there was really only one direction for him to roll and stumble as he tried to regain his equilibrium. Once he was close to fully recovered, most of the team departed, leaving a couple of experienced trackers to verify his complete anesthetic recovery.

Our New Year's Eve celebration was diminished by Graham's situation. Joliami's crushing bite had fortunately not injured any large blood vessels, but the damage to Graham's thigh was painful. Thanks to some strong pain-killers, though, he was quickly able to joke about the episode and to accept my apology for making a bad professional decision in darting Joliami from a dangerous position. Graham was back in the field in a few weeks, with just a slight lingering limp and a nice scar to show for his close call, while the hero of the day earned a new nickname, Super Barabwiriza.

Joliami's recovery was not as easy to monitor. As a lone silverback, no doubt intent on eluding anyone who might dart him again, he was hard to follow. But since he was also injured, his trackers were able to find him on most days and to verify that he was moving around a bit and managing to eat with only a little difficulty. They also observed him licking and cleaning but not chewing his wounds, which was good news to us.

On the sixth day after the intervention, Felicia and I made another visit with Barabwiriza. Joliami doubled back on his own trail and gave us the slip multiple times, which had us all laughing at being outsmarted by a gorilla, but eventually we tracked him back to his former group. This worried us at first, as it was possible he'd suffered his wounds at the hands of his own group members and that returning injured might invite another thorough beating. To our relief, the group members mostly ignored him, except for his younger brother, who greeted him and then spent time inspecting his wounds. We too had a good opportunity to assess them as Joliami sat quietly among his friends and family. His injuries were healing well, and it seemed likely that he would recover most of the use of his hands and go on to lead a normal life.

Unfortunately, no one has been able to verify Joliami's recovery, as he left the group shortly after that visit and hasn't been definitively seen since. We continue to hope that he will eventually turn up as the dominant silverback in a group. He was just approaching his physical prime, and it is common for lone silverbacks to elude observation for many years before starting or taking over their own groups, so we're still optimistic that this story about the big-eared gorilla will have a happy ending.

The flexible model Felicia and I created that day for working together during gorilla interventions went on to serve us well for many years. There were many occasions in which we had to go in separate directions or work on two gorillas in the same group—confirming that there was indeed enough work for two separate veterinarians. We continued to improve our field procedures during the succeeding years and worked together to train in-country veterinarians. No matter what issues we had with apportioning office and administrative work or with the other stresses of living and working in central Africa, we were always able to bring out the best in each other when a gorilla's health was on the line.

ABOUT THE AUTHORS

Christopher A. Whittier grew up on a small family farm in rural New Hampshire. He received double bachelor's degrees at Brown University, during which time he studied abroad in Tanzania. He also traveled across parts of east and central Africa, visiting many primate field sites. While earning his veterinary degree from Tufts University School of Veterinary Medicine, he returned to Tanzania to study the parasites of wild chimpanzees. Fascinated with primates, Dr. Whittier went on to work as relief veterinarian at the Duke Primate Center and began his PhD at North Carolina State University on the molecular diagnostics and epidemiology of diseases in wild gorillas. His graduate work led him back to Africa, this time to Rwanda. He and his wife, Felicia, worked together for several years as regional field veterinarians for the Mountain Gorilla Veterinary Project. The couple recently returned to the United States, and he is now finishing his dissertation.

Felicia B. Nutter announced when she was four years old that she was going to be a veterinarian, and went on to graduate from Tufts University School of Veterinary Medicine in 1993. Always interested in great apes, she studied parasites among chimpanzees, baboons, and humans at Gombe National Park, Tanzania, as a Fulbright fellow. Dr. Nutter returned to the United States for a small animal medicine and surgery internship, residency in zoological medicine (specializing in free-ranging wildlife), and PhD in population medicine, all at North Carolina State University College of Veterinary Medicine. She joined the Mountain Gorilla Veterinary Project in 2002, where she and Chris worked together for four years. Dr. Nutter became staff veterinarian for The Marine Mammal Center in Sausalito, California, in 2007, where she works with individual clinical cases, helps train young veterinarians, and studies health issues that impact the conservation of larger populations and entire species.

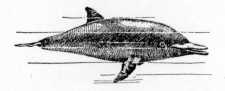

The Katrina Dolphins

by Pamela Govett, DVM

Thousands of feet above the ocean, I walked down the double row of blue and white fiberglass boxes lining the inside of the dimly lit DC-8, checking on the sixteen gray fusiform bodies that filled them. The dolphins, suspended in hammocks and resting in temperature-controlled water, seemed to be traveling comfortably. I was relieved. Outfitted in black rubber pants, a blue "Atlantis" T-shirt, and waterproof boots, I looked no different from the other specialists working with me. But they were seasoned veterans. This was my first dolphin transport.

The animals on the plane had quite a history. They had all been owned by the Marine Life Oceanarium, in Gulfport, Mississippi. In one way or another, each had lost its home on August 29, 2005, when Hurricane Katrina hit the

Gulf Coast. Thanks to the storm alerts, five of the dolphins at the Oceanarium were transferred to local hotel swimming pools to weather the storm. Another eight resident dolphins were placed in the Oceanarium's main pool, which had withstood previous hurricanes.

Unfortunately, the unusually large storm surge severely damaged the facility and swept the dolphins out to sea. Miraculously, all eight were rescued twelve days later by the Navy, and temporarily housed at the Gulfport, Mississippi naval base. The five that had endured the storm in hotel swimming pools found temporary homes at Florida's Gulfarium in Fort Walton Beach. The Oceanarium owned four additional dolphins that were on loan to various other institutions in the Northeast. They had been scheduled to return to Gulfport in the near future, and now they too were homeless.

Just prior to the hurricane, I had accepted a job at Atlantis resort in Nassau, Bahamas, as staff veterinarian. We were in the process of developing a brand-new, state-of-the-art facility for dolphins when Katrina hit. Atlantis offered the dolphins a home and Marine Life Oceanarium agreed. After the initial excitement, I found my new job turning into many late nights spent preparing for the dolphins' arrival. The health and welfare of the Katrina dolphins would soon be my responsibility, and I had to make sure that our facility contained everything they might need.

A top priority was to get to know the dolphins before we moved them to the Bahamas. That way, I'd be aware of their current health status and be able to detect a health problem early on. In the short month available to me before the move date, I visited as many of the aquaria and temporary facilities housing the dolphins as possible. I headed first to the naval base in Mississippi to meet the eight dolphins that had been swept out to sea three months earlier. Unused to fishing for themselves, the dolphins had lost noticeable weight and were in fragile condition at the time of their rescue. With the help of good nutrition and supportive care, they were now improving.

The day I arrived was cold and wet. Steady rain fell on the blue plastic roof of the warehouse where the dolphins had lived since the hurricane. As I stepped inside the shadowy, musty-smelling building, a cheery hello surprised me. The greeting came from one of the civilians employed to make sure the dolphins had clean artificial seawater in which to live. Enveloped in a large gray sweatshirt emblazoned "Navy" and sporting a blond braid down her back, the young woman was huddled by an electric heater. I shivered in my black Gore-Tex jacket and pulled it closer around me.

In a makeshift booth at one side of the vast building, the trainers were putting together the dolphins' meal of capelin and herring. I watched as they stuffed the fish with pills, hiding vitamins and medication deep inside where the dolphins wouldn't notice. Their haggard faces showed the strain of working long hours on behalf of the dolphins, with few days off. I wondered if part of their dedication to these animals was the shared experience of the hurricane; the trainers had lost their homes and belongings to the storm too.

There were two large collapsible pools in one corner of the warehouse, similar in size to the average backyard swimming pool. When the trainers approached the first pool, four surprisingly healthy-looking dolphins raised their heads out of the foamy water littered with play toys like hula hoops, plastic bats, and balls; they were eager for their next meal. Another four heads emerged for their fish in the second pool. The trainers introduced me to each one: Toni, Kelly, Tamra, Jill, Elijah, Noah, Jackie, and Michelle.

Though the warehouse itself felt gloomy, I could see the dolphins were well taken care of. I also knew they had a bright future. No expense had been spared during construction of their new home in Nassau, and the location was ideal—a lovely, warm vacation destination. The Atlantis facility included an acclimation habitat built on an intercoastal waterway and an inland permanent habitat. Each offered spacious open-water bedrooms and even larger interactive play areas. Water quality had been checked for the past year, and plans called for continued checks four times a week. Local fish schooled throughout the habitat, adding interest to the natural bottom that was meticulously scanned by snorkelers and divers to ensure that it was free of harmful debris.

The medical monitoring equipment was superior to that of most local hospitals. Blood samples could be analyzed in five minutes. Digital images of microscopic cells could be shared instantly with specialists hundreds of miles away. A hood and incubator had been installed so that the laboratory could perform its own microbiology work. An ultrasound unit the size of a waffle maker could be taken dockside to monitor pregnancies. The pharmacy contained all the medications the dolphins could ever need. The management plan focused on prevention: respirations, appetite, and attitude would be monitored daily, blood work and blowhole excretions routinely.

When I left the Mississippi warehouse that day, I felt bad

for the trainers. They would certainly miss these friendly and intelligent animals with whom they had developed such special bonds. With the departure of the dolphins, they would also have to find new jobs.

The next week, I flew to Florida to meet five more of the dolphins. I was able to spend two weeks with this group, and felt as though I got to know them well. There were two lively adolescents, Jonah and Brewer; a mother-and-daughter pair, Cherie and Katelyn; and an older female, Tessie. The trainers often played football and chase with Jonah and Katelyn after meals and daily exercises, and I jumped at the chance to join in. Assuming a more veterinary role, I examined the animals as they went through their husbandry routines. I consulted with the veterinarians who were in charge of their care at the time and pored over their medical records. I also helped prepare the transport containers.

Though I struggled not to show preference, Jonah quickly became my favorite. His upturned nose gave him a permanent cartoonish smile, and his impish ways and eagerness to interact with me, as well as with the other dolphins, made him irresistible. Brewer, a few years older than Jonah, had an entirely different personality, dutiful and eager to please. As for the females, the mother-and-daughter pair could not have been more different from each other. Sweet, graceful, and beautiful, Katelyn was endearing. Her mother, Cherie, had a devilish side.

Tessie was another story. Stricken by a rare fungal disease since the hurricane, she'd been fighting for her life. Only one other dolphin had been known to survive this type of infection, narrowly escaping death with the help of a new medication imported from Europe. During my brief visit in Florida, Tessie's condition had stabilized on this new medicine, but it was a struggle. The dedicated veterinary staff and trainers spent long hours coaxing Tessie to eat and accept her treatments. Fortunately, the fungus was not contagious to the other dolphins. Tessie was, technically, the seventeenth Katrina dolphin. Sadly, she was too ill to join the other sixteen on the flight to Nassau.

Two days before our flight to Nassau, I met the other four dolphins for the first time. I'd flown north to the National Aquarium in Baltimore to meet two males, Echo and Wee Tee, and participate in their move by truck to the airport. I'd spent only a short amount of time with this pair, but had been impressed by their alertness. Always on the lookout, ignoring each other but acutely aware of anything out of the ordinary, they would have made great espionage agents. Fortunate to have missed the hurricane, they'd been on loan to a Philadelphia aquarium when the storm hit; recently, they'd been moved to Baltimore.

The next day, I met the final two dolphins, Naia and Sasha, just as they were readied to board the plane. They'd been living at a New Jersey facility at the time of the hurricane. Since I'd had no chance to get to know them, I planned to spend extra time with them once we settled in at the new facility.

It had been a strenuous month for me, to put it mildly. In preparation for the move, I'd gone over every possible scenario in my mind. It's rare to transport so many dolphins at once, and a lot could go wrong. The animals might thrash around in their transport units, or breathe too rapidly due to stress. I was prepared to sedate them, but only if necessary.

The first step of the transport hadn't started off well at all. In Baltimore, Wee Tee and Echo were due to be moved onto a truck in late afternoon in preparation for the journey to the Philadelphia airport. Our trip out of Baltimore and into Philly had been carefully scheduled to occur at night, to avoid high traffic both on the streets and at the airport. But the pump in the dolphins' pool malfunctioned; we were unable to lower the water enough so that we could glide the dolphins into their transport hammocks. Eventually, the maintenance staff fixed the problem, but the delay threatened to disrupt our precise schedule.

With the pool drained, I watched anxiously as the trainers positioned Echo into his hammock first, followed by Wee Tee. A pulley system lifted both hammocks out of the pool and a digital scale measured their weights: 450 pounds for Echo and 400 for Wee Tee. The dolphins appeared calm, though they must have been acutely aware that everything around them was changing. Once loaded onto a twenty-four-foot rental truck, the hammocks were suspended inside special individual transportation units filled with water kept at a cozy 76° Fahrenheit. Finally I had something to do that would directly benefit my patients: before we drove off into the chill night air, I liberally rubbed vitamin A and D ointment onto the dolphins' bodies to help prevent chafing and desiccation.

While a team of police officers on motorcycles led us through busy city streets, I kept my focus on the dolphins. Thankfully, the dolphin team included four other people who'd done this many times before. Together we monitored the dolphins' respirations, heart rate, and demeanor. At one point, the truck screeched abruptly to a stop, and a wave of water swelled up and out of the transport boxes, all over me. Drenched, I burst into surprised laughter. I thought maybe this was like a wedding where there's always one thing that isn't quite perfect. I decided it was fine with me if my getting soaked turned out to be that one thing.

At the Philadelphia airport, things went much more smoothly. We met up as planned with the other transport team from New Jersey, and I had time to check briefly on Sasha and Naia. I climbed into the back of the truck and spent a few minutes with each. Sasha, an adult female, looked a bit on the plump side. Naia, a youngster, had beautiful brown eyes. Both appeared to be doing well.

All four dolphins were quickly loaded on the cargo plane that would fly us all to Nassau via the Mobile airport, where the other twelve dolphins had already arrived. The logistics team did a terrific job, and even though it was the middle of the night, the rendezvous went perfectly. Before long, we took off again with all sixteen dolphins on board, scheduled to arrive in Nassau at sunrise.

—

During the brief flight, I thought again about recent events. On one hand, these were lucky dolphins indeed. On the other hand, I felt sad for their trainers and for the many people in Mississippi who'd helped with the amazing rescue of the dolphins. It must have been very difficult for them to say good-bye. I also knew that not everyone agreed on the move—or the sale—of the animals to the resort. But it would have been years before the dolphins could live together again as a group, since their hurricane-damaged facility had to be completely rebuilt, at a time when funds and energy were desperately needed for relief of the human devastation caused by Katrina.

Though everything had gone well so far, my stomach felt tight. I kept fiddling with the elastic band in my hair, which was tied in a ponytail to keep it from falling in my face. I wanted no distractions as I worked my way to the back of the plane, stopping to check each dolphin. Toni, an inquisitive adult female, lifted her head as if to greet me. I smiled as I patted her and whispered, "Hello." She nestled back down into her hammock. Next I came to Kelly, who seemed to be whistling in conversation with Tamra in the carrier next to her. These were among the dolphins that had been swept out to sea, and yet they looked almost unscathed. As the plane continued to jet southward in the early morning hours, the only visible reminder of their struggle to survive was a tear in Toni's dorsal fin.

Reaching the back of the plane, I stopped to check on Echo and Wee Tee, resting peacefully, seemingly unfazed by the events of the day. With a flashlight, I peered down their blowholes to study the color and pattern of their mucous membranes, the characteristics of their eyes, individual markings—anything that might help me to be a better doctor to them. It would take years for me to develop the kind of relationship I'd seen in Florida between Tessie and the park staff, but this was a start.

As we landed, the water shifted in the dolphin carriers. Miraculously, not a drop spilled. We gathered up our equipment, readied our packs, and stretched our stiff bodies.

When the airplane cargo door glided open, the interior lights also went on. I squinted in the harsh gleam, trying to adjust to the fact that we'd actually arrived. Into the plane stepped members of the Department of Agriculture, along with the president of Atlantis resort. We excitedly introduced them to our precious cargo.

I poked my head out the doorway and saw that a crowd of more than 150 people had come to welcome the dolphins at this predawn hour. The warm, moist air felt soft and comforting on my tired face. One by one, the dolphins were loaded off the plane to applause and expressions of joy. A forklift loaded the transportation units onto four flatbed trucks. As the sun rose, we went rolling down the streets of Nassau. Although it was now a busy time of morning in town, the military escorts provided by the city carried out their job perfectly. We seemed to reach our destination in no time. These sixteen new residents were obviously very special to the Bahamians!

When we came to a stop outside the dolphins' new home, a crane appeared and gently lifted the hammocks from the transportation units. The dolphins were carried by teams of ten people down to their new open-air holding pools, filled with beautiful blue Caribbean water. Each animal was set gently along the edge of the dock, with the pectoral fin nearest the water tucked beside its body. Someone called, "One . . . two . . . three . . . GO!" and the dolphins were carefully rolled out of the hammocks and into the water.

The dolphins' response amazed me. I'd seen these animals swimming quietly or simply resting in their various temporary homes. Here, they immediately began leaping in and out of the water, occasionally chasing small fish, rolling over one another in play. Never had I seen them so active!

I smiled with a sense of accomplishment as I sat on the dock and watched the dolphins convene. The adrenaline that had been coursing through my body was waning and the effects of being awake for thirty-six hours were beginning to take their toll. "Welcome to your new home, beautiful dolphins," I said.

ABOUT THE AUTHOR

Pamela Govett has long held an interest in ocean life and began her career researching cetacean vocalizations. She received her veterinary degree at the University of Florida, after which she completed an internship in small animal medicine and surgery at the University of Georgia. Next came a residency in zoo, wildlife, and aquatic animal medicine at North Carolina State University, followed by a position as interim associate veterinarian at the New England Aquarium in Boston. She served as head veterinarian at Atlantis resort in Paradise Island, Bahamas, where she looked after not only dolphins, but sea turtles, sharks, rays, fish, and birds. Dr. Govett is currently an assistant professor at Western University College of Veterinary Medicine in Pomona, California.

IV

PUZZLES AND MYSTERIES

Despite their years of special training, zoo vets are acutely aware of what they don't know. Most of us keep a library of textbooks and subscribe to reference material on the Internet on topics ranging from domestic and wild animal medicine to emerging infectious diseases and human pediatrics. We also publish what we learn from clinical practice and applied research, adding to the growing annals of zoological animal medicine. When strange cases arise, as they often do, we call our colleagues and other experts for ideas.

Solving medical problems in any species is analogous to putting together a difficult puzzle without all the pieces. Though the reference literature grows by the year, zoo vets confronted by a mystery often must rely on hunches backed up by personal experience, ingenuity, and patience.

The animal's clinical signs are important clues. Some injuries are obvious, like a bleeding wound or broken leg. But trauma to muscles or internal organs may not be evident from a distance, or even in the animal's overall behavior. And nervous animals can often override pain. An anxious impala may run on a sore foot as if nothing were wrong. Signs of illness can be equally obscure. A wolf with a liver problem and a history of vomiting may keep its food down at one meal, but not the next. Sometimes it's what an animal doesn't do that gives cause for worry. A chimpanzee known for his feisty behavior is not feeling 100 percent if he misses an opportunity to spit a mouthful of water at the vet.

As the basis for interpreting an animal's behavior as abnormal, zoo vets also need to know the biology of the species concerned. The animal's natural history—its preferred habitat and diet, its reproductive cycle—influences how well it takes medicine or tolerates anesthesia and hospitalization. Certain species, especially nervous or social ones like birds, hoofed animals, and primates, can develop entirely new problems associated with the stress of treatment.

Once we've done a hands-on physical exam and run various laboratory tests, we check our results against previously established baseline data for that species. Sometimes that information may turn out not to be very useful. For example, published normal results for a complete blood count, or CBC, in a golden monkey might be based on a handful of animals, some living in captivity, others free-living. With such a small sample size, it's impossible to distinguish subtle differences between the results for individuals of different ages and sex. Some variation may be entirely normal. By contrast, baseline data for these tests in humans and domestic animals is widely available and based on huge sample sizes.

With the data gathered, we try to put the pieces of the puzzle together. We can usually pinpoint the problem to a particular body system. As in any species, there are only so many: cardiac, respiratory, digestive, nervous, immune, reproductive, urinary, and musculoskeletal. But certain diseases, like cancer and nutritional imbalances, affect the whole animal.

Like all doctors, zoo vets prefer to base their therapy on a specific diagnosis. But while tests are pending, our patient may be suffering. If we think we can help the animal feel better, without doing harm, we will prescribe nonspecific treatment, or perhaps treat for the most likely problem. The patient's response to therapy often helps us to confirm or refute our best-guess diagnosis. Sometimes the definitive test result comes in long after the animal has healed.

But as the stories in this section show, some puzzles elude solution—at least in the beginning. Others are solved in time to save the patient. And some, to our great frustration, remain unsolved. The patients here include a Bengal tiger, a giant Pacific octopus, a white rhino, a group of dung beetles, a red-ruffed lemur, and a Pacific bottlenose dolphin.

Lucy H. Spelman, DVM

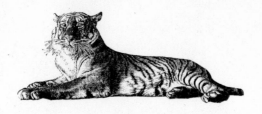

The Limping Tiger

by David Taylor, BVMS

> Tiger! Tiger! Burning bright
> In the forests of the night,
> What immortal hand or eye
> Could frame thy fearful symmetry?
> —William Blake, "The Tiger"

Zelda, the Bengal tigress at Windsor Safari Park in the UK, was not displaying much fearful symmetry. She padded unsteadily across the green sward of the reserve where she and twelve of her fellow tigers lived. I stood next to Ginger, the highly experienced ex–circus man in charge of the park's big-cat collection.

"It beats me," he said. "Fit as a fiddle two days ago. Look at her now! I put her in a small cage this morning and checked her legs. Nothing amiss that I could see. No bite wounds, no overgrown claws pricking her foot pads." He shook his head slowly. Zelda was Ginger's particular favorite. He had helped me deliver her when her mother had difficulty giving birth six years earlier, in 1982.

"Let's get her inside," I replied. "We'll have a proper look at her under anesthesia."

By gently guiding her with a Land Rover, Ginger and his men persuaded Zelda to go into her night-house. I used my dart pistol to inject her with a light dose of ketamine, a short-acting anesthetic.

Five minutes after the flying dart hit her rump, she was asleep. We could safely enter her quarters. Ginger unlocked the door and I went in. (I have always made a point of being the first to enter when a potentially dangerous beast has been sedated. Since the vet picks the drug and the dose, he or she should take responsibility for the initial close encounter with the animal—just in case it isn't drowsing quite as deeply as it might appear.)

I knelt beside this most magnificent of cats as she lay on her side, resting on a bed of wooden railroad ties covered with a layer of straw. I checked her heart and lungs with my stethoscope and took her pulse by feeling beneath her upper-most hind leg for the femoral artery. All fine. I reckoned I had about ten minutes before she began to rouse significantly. I ran my fingers over her limbs. I could find nothing wrong with her great paws, nor were there any abnormal swellings along the long bones of her legs. One by one, I felt her joints, moving and gently pinching them. Was their movement smooth? Could I feel any loss of fluidity, any "scrunching" sensation of bone rubbing against bone? Were the ones on her right side the same size and shape as those on her left?

I soon felt something. One—nay, both—of her knee joints were puffier than normal. Then I got the impression that one hock (ankle) joint and both the carpal (wrist) joints of her forelegs were enlarged. I could feel extra fluid under pressure between the adjoining bones.

"What do you think, Doc?" whispered Ginger, kneeling beside me.

"Joints for sure," I replied, "but what exactly I don't know. Could be arthritis, perhaps caused by a bacterial infection. Never seen anything quite like it in big cats before."

On occasion, I had dealt with cases of multiple joint inflammation, or polyarthritis, in other species. We had a case in a giraffe, also at Windsor, that we ended up treating with acupuncture. But I had never heard of it in big cats in zoos or circuses. I decided to give Zelda a course of antibiotics together with anti-inflammatory corticosteroid drugs. We gave this to her by injection and planned to continue dosing her in her food.

"I'll come back to see her again in five days."

The telephone rang early next morning. It was Ginger reporting that Zelda's condition had worsened markedly. She could barely walk and was unable to leave the night-house. I set off at once for the safari park. As I drove, I puzzled over the tigress's condition. She wasn't old, so age-related osteoarthritis seemed unlikely. Could it be septic arthritis caused by bacteria arriving via the bloodstream? Possible, but I'd never seen or heard of such a condition in big cats. What to do? Radiography perhaps. Draw off a sample of what might well be purulent joint fluid for bacteriological culture? Probably the best course. Treatment? For the moment at least continue antibiotics, switch from corticosteroids to nonsteroidal anti-inflammatory drugs until I had a precise diagnosis. Certainly, I had to relieve Zelda's pain as a priority.

Ginger was waiting by the tiger area gate when I arrived. "She's bad, Doc," he said as we walked to the night-houses. "An' on top of her lameness, her appetite's gone and bless me if her eyes aren't changing color!"

"What do you mean?" I asked, eyebrows raised.

"The shine has gone; they're dark-colored now." He muttered an oath under his breath.

The tigress lay awkwardly on her bedding. The swollen joints were now plain to see and, yes, her eyes did appear to have changed color. I immediately set about preparing a flying dart and filling it with ketamine. The cat managed a growl of protest when the dart hit her.

As soon as she was drowsing peacefully, I began by inspecting her head with the apparently color-changed eyes. Looking closely, I confirmed what Ginger had described. Her eyes were indeed darker. The effect was caused by an accumulation of dark blood in the anterior chamber, between the front of the iris and the back of the cornea, of each eye. This was something I had never seen before in any species of cat—hyphema, bleeding within the eye.

Next, I turned to the puffy joints. After shaving and disinfecting a small area of skin over one hock, I passed a sterile hypodermic needle into the enlarged joint cavity and attached a syringe. Pulling back the plunger, I waited for fluid to emerge. Straightaway it did. Within a couple of seconds, I had a syringe full of pure blood. Oh Lord, I thought, blood in the eyes, blood in the joints, blood perhaps leaking elsewhere in the body. I think I know what this might be.

Ginger saw the worried expression on my face. A small tear glistened on his cheek. This burly, chain-smoking, beer-loving, three-fry-ups-a-day head keeper—who knew more about the ways of big cats than any other animal man I had ever worked with—understood Zelda was in trouble.

"T'aint serious, is it, Doc?" he murmured. "Arthritis can't kill, can it?"

"I'm afraid it *is* serious, Ginger," I replied. "If I'm right, Zelda has been poisoned."

There was a long pause before my companion spoke again. "Poisoned? By what? How? Who by?"

"A chemical that stops blood clotting. The most likely culprit is the rodent poison coumarin, better known as warfarin. Kills rats and mice by causing them to hemorrhage internally. Sometimes happens in domestic animals that eat rat poison, though I've never seen it in exotic cats. Are you using warfarin to control pests in the reserve?" I knew that the stuff was sometimes used in zoos to get rid of rodents.

"Warfarin. Yes, it's used by the pest control firm that the park contracts, but it's never put down in bait boxes inside the reserves, only outside where our animals couldn't get at it."

"Do you ever see rats in the reserves?"

"Occasionally. I've seen tigers, lions, and cheetahs sometimes chasing one."

"And catching and eating it?"

Ginger thought for a moment and then said, "I have seen it happen."

I decided to take a blood sample from Zelda while she still slept and send it to the local laboratory. The key test I wanted to run was called a prothrombin time, a measure of blood coagulation time. My problem now was that although I knew what a normal prothrombin time should be for humans and domestic cats (both the same, between eleven and fourteen seconds), I had no idea what it should be for tigers.

"Let's drive round the reserve and see if all the other cats seem okay. I'll also knock out Zeinab, Zelda's mother, so I can take a blood sample from her for comparison." As we left Zelda's night-house I saw her pass a little urine; it was the color of rosé wine.

All of the other tigers seemed perfectly healthy. Using my telescopic dart rifle, I injected Zeinab's shoulder and within a few minutes had the necessary blood. While the two samples were sent to the lab, I called the big-cat keepers together and explained what I thought had happened.

"An animal doesn't have to eat warfarin itself to be poisoned. It can also happen if it eats an animal that already is suffering or dead from consuming warfarin. Usually for poisoning to happen, the warfarin has to be ingested on several occasions, but some species can be affected after a single dose. We just don't know how sensitive tigers are. Have any of you guys seen rats inside the tiger reserve?" I asked.

Several of the men nodded at once.

One keeper said, "Actually I saw Zelda chasing a rat, killing it, and eating it a few days ago. She didn't have to make much of an effort. It was walking slowly and staggering a bit across some short grass."

Here was a highly plausible explanation for how Zelda became sickened by warfarin. A rat eats the poison bait outside the tiger reserve, falls ill, and, when close to death, goes blindly through the chain-link fence and wobbles its way into the jaws of the tigress.

Within an hour, the laboratory rang. Zelda's prothrombin time was fifty-five seconds; her mother's blood coagulated normally in twelve seconds. I was now certain that the tigress was poisoned by warfarin.

Warfarin achieves its toxic effect by attacking vitamin K, an essential component of the blood-clotting mechanism. Treatment for Zelda meant big doses of vitamin K for the next few days at least. We put an urgent call to the pharmaceutical wholesalers for a courier to be sent to the park at once, bringing more vitamin K injectable solution than I'd ever used in my whole career.

By this time, Zelda had come round from the anesthetic, so I gave her the first dose by flying dart from a blowpipe. Later that day I repeated the procedure.

Within twenty-four hours, there was a noticeable improvement in the tigress. She could rise to her feet and walk with less difficulty. Twice a day for the next week, I gave her more vitamin K by blow dart. By the third day, her eyes were back to their usual appearance of burnished gold. The blood in the anterior chamber gradually reabsorbed. The color of her urine also returned to normal, clear yellow, and so did her appetite.

Ten days later, the joint swellings had fully resolved and Zelda could walk, run, and spring with her usual elegant fluidity. Another prothrombin test gave us a gratifying reading of fifteen.

Ginger and I went to the pub in Windsor to celebrate Zelda's recovery. Warfarin would no longer be used by the rodent controllers at the safari park, he informed me. I announced that I'd be presenting the park with a pair of Lancashire heelers, the best little ratting dogs I'd ever come across.

Soon the dogs joined the safari park staff and began patrolling the grounds with the security men during the night. Rats were never much of a problem in Windsor Safari Park from then on. Zelda herself went on to have several litters of fine cubs.

Sadly, the safari park closed several years later. I bumped into Ginger while walking through Windsor. We talked about his tigers, which had been relocated to parks in the English Midlands.

"Went to see old Zelda a couple of weeks ago," he told me. "She's in fine fettle. But I'll tell you what, Doc, we should all keep away from hospitals. These physicians are a dangerous lot! My pal's had heart trouble and the quacks wanted to put him on warfarin—same stuff as poisoned Zelda!"

I reassured my friend that the infamous rat poison was nowadays being used as a lifesaving anticoagulant in the blood of human patients. Ginger looked doubtful. On that note, we adjourned to the pub.

ABOUT THE AUTHOR

David Taylor received his veterinary degree from the University of Glasgow Veterinary School in 1956 and was appointed a fellow of the Royal College of Veterinary Surgeons in Diseases of Zoo Primates in 1968. He founded the International Zoo Veterinary Group in 1969 and has worked in countries all over the world. In recent years, Dr. Taylor has specialized in marine mammal medicine. He is also the author of some fifty books on animal matters, including seven autobiographical volumes in the *Zoovet* series. He is married with two daughters and lives just outside of London.

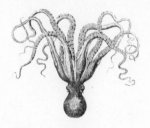

Sliced Bananas in Jell-O

by Michael Stoskopf, DVM, PhD

W hen did it start?"

"I don't know for sure. Two weeks ago she was a bit slower to come out. Not as aggressive as usual. Now she isn't eating at all. Is it happening already?"

"I hope not. It shouldn't be. She isn't that big yet, but this is how they say it starts. The whole thing doesn't make much sense to me."

"To me either, Doc, but they sure are delicate. We've had Bertha months longer than any of the others, and everyone says they only live three years. When she got to Baltimore last year [1984], I'm sure she had to be at least a year old. They don't grow very fast when they are here. I'm guessing she is between two and three years old."

"I don't get it either, Doug, the whole thing is strange.

Endocrine glands suddenly enlarging beside the optic nerves, and then—instant senility. It doesn't seem right. I know nature is stranger than fiction, but I'm not sure I can buy into such a large and intelligent animal being essentially disposable. They have to live longer in the wild. Besides, the first ones we had arrived nearly dead, did poorly in our water, or injured themselves escaping. We've only seen the large optic glands on one animal, Ollie, and he was a male, and much larger than Bertha. Maybe the glands aren't the issue at all."

"Maybe, Doc. I hope you're right, but what do we do with Bertha?"

While we talked, Doug, the senior aquarist in charge of the octopus gallery, didn't break his steady observations of the giant Pacific octopus, Bertha. Bertha sat holed up in her favorite large broken crock, holding herself in position with her large suckered tentacles. Her expiratory siphons moved rhythmically, bringing oxygenated water past her gills. Her color was a vibrant mottled red with black patterns, a good sign. The earlier animals had become pale a few weeks before their deaths. There also was no evidence that Bertha was picking at herself—yet. We had watched Bertha's predecessor, Ollie, pull at his own flesh, creating large irregular ulcers on his mantle. A few weeks later he finally died, despite our best efforts to treat the wounds.

If it weren't for Doug's intense familiarity with Bertha's moods and habits, no one would suspect anything was wrong with her. Maybe it was something simple like indigestion, and not the fatal octopus endocrine senility syndrome. I'd found this strange syndrome described in a fifteen-year-old article in *Science* magazine. But if Bertha's problem wasn't senility, what was it? How could we find out what the problem was?

The aquarium had struggled to learn how to house these big, intelligent invertebrate animals. First there were the shipment problems. The very large wild-caught specimens didn't do well on cross-country trips from their northern Pacific range, even when shipped inside specially designed high-tech life-support barrels. If your aquarium wasn't on the West Coast, then catching and shipping smaller animals was the only answer. Unfortunately, octopi that arrived in good condition then proved capable of escaping from the exhibit with impunity.

They could maneuver through unbelievably small cracks between the heaviest tank lids and the exhibit walls. Once out of the exhibit, they'd be stranded on the floor behind the exhibit, without access to saltwater. Though the escaped animals would be found alive when the aquarists came in early in the morning, they never fared well afterward. When heavier lids on the exhibit didn't solve the problem, we lined the top of the exhibit with artificial turf, a plastic material that prevents the eight-tentacled, Houdini-like animals from attaching their powerful suckers to gain purchase to allow them to squeeze under the display lids.

The escapees taught us something else. Sometimes it was hard to tell if the octopus was alive. One of the first animals to escape was found lying apparently lifeless on the floor in a back room near its tank. The octopus was pronounced dead and delivered in a sealed plastic bag to the pathologists at the university. But when the pathologist took the supposedly dead animal out of the refrigerator and started to prepare for the necropsy examination, the octopus reached up and grabbed the arm of the startled scientist. A police car, sirens blaring, escorted the animal back through the city to the aquarium. Sadly, several days of supportive care, monitoring, and all of our efforts to revive the animal met with no success. But I did learn a great deal about octopi in the process, like how to take a blood sample and how to read an octopus EKG.

At first glance no one would think of Bertha as delicate. However, like other cephalopods, giant Pacific octopi are very sensitive to tiny amounts of toxic metals and slight imbalances of essential elements in their water. And the water must be cold. Facilities successfully keeping these animals alive for long periods in the past all had natural seawater pumped into their exhibits, an advantage we didn't enjoy. Keeping giant octopi healthy with artificially made seawater posed many unexplored challenges. Water that is perfectly suitable even for delicate corals, another type of aquatic invertebrate, can prove problematic for an octopus. There's also the difficulty that when octopi become agitated, they release a dark plume of chemicals popularly known as ink. In the wild, an octopus uses this discharge to befuddle prey or to serve as a distraction while escaping its own predators. The ink contains several neuroactive compounds that cause disorientation and confusion. An octopus in the wild would normally move rapidly away from an area it had inked to avoid being affected. In the exhibit tank, of course, that isn't possible.

Fortunately, Doug had been able to solve the water issues. He was one of those people who just seem to have a "green thumb" with delicate marine creatures. It wasn't simply his careful attention to detail, or his deep curiosity about the animals, it was also a gift for understanding the needs of his animals that every great aquarist or zookeeper seems to have. Thanks to many expensive sophisticated water tests, Doug found and removed all sources of heavy metals from the exhibit and refined the artificial seawater mix. He also figured out ways to reduce the anxiety caused in these intelligent animals due to their being on public display by giving them better hiding places and more things to manipulate, and lowering the light levels in the gallery. This effectively reduced the risk of an inking event. These advances had allowed Bertha to live longer than the octopi before her, and long enough for us to suspect the rapid senility syndrome that we had first learned about while trying to save our previous giant Pacific octopus, Ollie.

Ollie had survived the early adjustments and lived apparently comfortably in his exhibit for nearly a year before he suddenly stopped eating. He then became listless, tearing at himself and opening the wounds we weren't able to heal. We made a number of advances in octopus medicine while trying to diagnose and treat Ollie, just not enough of them.

In veterinary medicine, blood samples often help us make a diagnosis, and I take pride in being able to get blood from even the most challenging of patients. I had figured out how to draw a blood sample from an octopus using landmarks I noted while dissecting the bodies of the less fortunate earlier animals in our collection. To take a sample from Ollie, one aquarist would hold on to a tentacle and pull it out of the water, while another tried to keep the animal from climbing up and biting with his strong beak, which is capable of cracking a crab shell with ease. When I inserted a needle directly into the vein supplying the tentacle, I could withdraw several milliliters of clear, slightly bluish blood. In relative terms, getting a blood sample wasn't that hard. Unfortunately, the analyses weren't very informative. No one had published what the blood of a normal giant Pacific octopus should look like. Nor was there any obvious pattern of change in the chemical composition or cell types when comparing the samples taken over the many weeks that Ollie refused to feed.

As his condition deteriorated, I found an article published many years before in the journal *Science* about a smaller species of tropical octopus being used in research. The paper described two large orange glands adjacent to the optic nerves that appeared just as the smaller octopi reached sexual maturity. If the glands were removed surgically, the article reported, the octopi could be induced to live longer and survive the reproductive stage of their lives. When Ollie died, we found those orange glands at the necropsy. We hadn't seen them in any of our earlier animals.

Could surgical removal of those glands save Bertha, or at least extend her life? Normally I'm willing to try radical measures to help a patient in crisis, but I hesitated to perform what amounted to delicate brain surgery on an animal whose illness consisted, so far, of missing a few meals. Besides, I had my own doubts about the supposedly "lethal" nature of the orange optic glands, despite the prestige of the journal *Science*. It seemed unlikely that this large, magnificent, and intelligent animal should be doomed to a single reproductive cycle and then senescent death.

On the other hand, I wasn't going to simply watch and wait. When working with any new species, my instincts tell me it is better to get on the case sooner rather than later. Bertha continued to refuse her crabs and any other tasty treat Doug could find to tempt her. Were her optic glands in fact enlarged? It was time for some creative diagnostic testing like octopus radiography to try to see the glands.

It wouldn't be easy. As far as I knew, no one had ever tried to anesthetize and position a thirty-five-pound water-breathing mass of muscle and intellect for an X-ray. The aquarium's small portable X-ray unit wouldn't be able to penetrate Bertha's body mass and give us the detail we would need to see if the glands were enlarged. That's why having a faculty appointment in the radiology department of a world-class medical school comes in handy. Time to call my friend Elliot and arrange for a CT scan.

Tall and blond, with a bristling mustache and dark-rimmed glasses framing his face, Elliot always seems to be in motion. While nurses and technicians efficiently put his human patients into the CT machine and generate images at a dizzying pace, Elliot choreographs it all and dictates incessantly into his recorder, interpreting the images and making life-impacting diagnoses. He is amazingly skilled but, more important, he is curious, and always makes time for my non-human patients. And his CT machine is fast. We would only need to keep Bertha still for a few minutes to collect many images of her.

I had learned a valuable lesson that would help me safely anesthetize Bertha from the wild ambulance return of the not-yet-dead octopus years ago. To protect the expensive CT equipment, we would anesthetize Bertha lightly, just to the point where she could no longer grab with her eight arms. Then we would put her in a plastic bag with some water, place her in the scanner, and quickly acquire images of her head region. Special software that Elliot and his research team had developed would allow us to reconstruct the images into a three-dimensional view. This would compensate for our inability to position Bertha precisely.

Over a period of nearly thirty minutes, we carefully induced Bertha's anesthesia. Then it was splash, zip, zap, and we had the images. Helping my technicians to extricate Bertha from her bag, I called to Elliot, "What do you see?"

"A bag full of Jell-O with banana slices all through it," Elliot called out over the intercom.

Sure enough, the CT scanner, which is very good at many things, didn't find enough differences in the density of Bertha's tissues to make useful images. Her powerful, muscular suckers showed up like big slices of bananas against a uniform gray background. Only her strong beak was discernible. We would have to try something else, maybe MRI—magnetic resonance imaging. MRI works on an entirely different principle than X-rays or CT scans, and provides a much better view of soft tissue structures. But it takes longer to make the images, and Bertha could not move during the imaging. Bertha would have to be under anesthesia for a longer time.

The challenges of applying MRI technology to an octopus might have been more intimidating, but for years I had been a member of the research team that was developing better methods of using the big magnets for diagnosing a wide range of conditions in humans and in animals. I knew the images we could obtain with the equipment would be far better for what we needed to see than CT, but I worried about subjecting Bertha to the longer and deeper anesthesia we would need to get those images. I had hoped the faster CT would do the job. Should we just take Bertha back to the aquarium and watch her behavior? Or should we try to keep her anesthetized in the bag long enough for an MRI?

Blackie, my wiry and very humorous British teammate on the MRI group, made the call. "Aw right now, in she goes, where she stops nobody knows. Just don't spill any water on me magnet."

Back into the bag went Bertha, this time with a bit more water. Blackie wasn't kidding. Any spill would ruin the multi-million-dollar research instrument. On top of that, the saltwater would dampen the signals in the machine. Luckily, our MRI development team had done something like this before. To improve the image quality for marine creatures, we'd built several special acquisition coils to collect signals from other animals that lived in saltwater. (They don't teach you this stuff in veterinary school!)

Blackie ran the instrument with skill and speed, as always. He initiated the data collection sequence almost before we could set Bertha on the gantry. As soon as we had data from the region between Bertha's eyes where we hoped to see the glands, I had her out of her bag and back in her traveling barrel.

Good news: Bertha hadn't moved, and we'd gotten good images. There were no signs of enlargement along the optic nerves. We could see these structures running from the

backs of her eyes and into her brain. There would be no reason to perform brain surgery on our girl, which made me
very happy. The bad news was that we were no closer to understanding why she wasn't eating.

After an uneventful ride back to the aquarium, sans sirens,
Bertha, still a bit groggy from her double bag experience,
slid into her exhibit and bunched herself up in her broken-
crockery hiding spot. A few days later, while we were making
our weekly medical rounds past the octopus exhibit, Doug
offered Bertha a delectable small blue crab. The crab had
barely taken two steps sideways after drifting to the bottom
of the exhibit before Bertha unexpectedly zoomed out of her
crock, engulfed the crab in her tentacles, and began to feed.
We joked that maybe the powerful magnet had realigned her
appetite, or that somehow the two anesthesia events had
calmed her nerves, but the most likely explanation was that
she had managed to get over a mild digestive upset on her
own with no help from us. Bertha continued to feed and
thrived under Doug's care for almost another year without
any signs of rapid senility syndrome. Unfortunately, she
eventually died from a rapidly progressing bacterial infection.

The quest to successfully maintain giant octopi and rear
them in captivity continues today. Several years after Bertha's
adventures, my suspicions were supported by important discoveries made by marine biologists working with these animals in the wild. We now know that their life span is much
greater than three years. Scientists continue to conduct interesting research about the lives of giant octopi in the cold wa-
ters of the Pacific Northwest. As we learn more about these

fascinating creatures, we find new ways to help them live longer and better lives in captivity, ensuring that they remain a part of our world for a long time to come.

ABOUT THE AUTHOR

Michael K. Stoskopf is a professor at North Carolina State University. He received his veterinary degree from Colorado State University, earned a PhD in toxicology from Johns Hopkins University, and is a diplomate in the American College of Zoological Medicine. In the course of his varied career, Dr. Stoskopf has run an unusual ambulatory practice in the mountains of Colorado, served as the veterinarian for the Overton Park Zoo in Memphis and the Baltimore Zoo, and taught on the faculty of the Johns Hopkins School of Medicine. He was the founding chief of medicine for the National Aquarium in Baltimore before taking on the challenges of teaching at a veterinary college. He and his wife, Dr. Suzanne Kennedy-Stoskopf, live on a small farm outside Raleigh, North Carolina, where they devote much of their energy to providing the next generation of veterinarians the knowledge and the skills necessary to make the world a better place for wildlife, people, and their domestic animals.

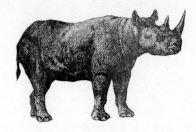

On the Horn of a Dilemma

by Steve Osofsky, DVM

I trained intensively to become a wildlife veterinarian in Africa—something I'd wanted to be for as long as I can remember, back to the time when I was six or seven years old watching (the original) Mutual of Omaha's *Wild Kingdom*. After veterinary school, I had purposely sought out a small animal internship in medicine and surgery in order to help me reinforce the top-notch way of doing everything. I wanted to make sure that when I did find myself out in remote bush someday, I'd be able to extrapolate and do my best with locally available materials.

When the government of Botswana hired me in 1991 to establish the Department of Wildlife and National Parks (DWNP) Wildlife Veterinary Unit, my childhood dream became a reality. At the same time, Botswana increased its

efforts to curtail poaching. A new Anti-Poaching Unit had begun to patrol remote areas of northern Botswana. These
long-overdue forays into the bush firmly established that rhinos had for years been slaughtered for their horns. Botswana
was on the verge of losing all of its white rhinos—again.

Between 1967 and 1982, South Africa had helped restock
Botswana's then poacher-depleted rhino population by
translocating ninety-four animals into protected areas in the
northern part of the country. Had these rhinos been adequately protected from that time on, there indeed should
have been *hundreds* in the wild by the early 1990s. But new
surveys revealed evidence of *only seven white rhinos.* Twelve
poached carcasses were identified in 1992 alone. By 1993,
emergency measures were clearly required.

In an all-out effort, a group of concerned citizens in the
large town of Serowe (birthplace of Sir Seretse Khama, the
beloved first president of Botswana) established the Khama
Rhino Sanctuary in close collaboration with the DWNP.
Located in the central part of the country, far from the
poaching threat in the north, the locally managed sanctuary
would provide the land, staff housing, and care for any rhinos
that had to be brought into captivity to protect them. While
several of us in the DWNP would provide the logistics support for capture, we didn't have the experience or equipment to carry out such a massive operation alone.

At my urging, the Botswana DWNP asked South Africa's
Natal Parks Board Rhino Capture Team to assist us. We had
two goals: to save the remaining white rhinos (and any black
rhinos we might find), and to train a DWNP team in the challenging art and science of rhino capture and translocation.

The middle of the rainy season is the worst time of the year to be hauling heavy trucks through the bush and mud. Of course, this was when we found three sets of rhino tracks leading to two rhinos—a cow and a calf shot dead by poachers. From the tracks, it looked as if one rhino had gotten away. With little time left to save the country's last wild rhinos, the DWNP's Cessna went out on reconnaissance.

On February 12, a rhino and calf in thick bush were spotted from the plane. The helicopter with the darting team was quickly guided into the area, and the capture trucks headed to a feasible rendezvous point. Radios crackled and tree branches cracked as the ground team rushed to the coordinates called out from the aircraft. Anesthetic darts shot from the helicopter found their marks: a thirty-year-old cow and her nine-month-old calf. The animals were successfully loaded into special rhino crates brought in from South Africa, and transported to the sanctuary *bomas* (pens) in Serowe.

That same day, another adult white rhino, an approximately thirty-year-old bull, was also darted, crated, and driven the fourteen hours to Serowe. Both the cow and bull had notched ears; the bull also sported a hole from an old ear tag. These ID markers meant that these animals were part of the group originally translocated from South Africa at least a decade ago. How sad that they now needed to be saved—but how honored we were to do it. I sawed off the big bull's horn before we crated him, and we made sure the word got out that there would be no horns for the picking in Serowe. A rhino's horn, like one's fingernails, slowly grows back. This was the safest approach for all concerned.

On February 15, a three- to four-year-old bull was found wandering on his own about twenty kilometers from where the other animals had been caught. Once we'd darted him and were able to give him a thorough hands-on exam, I saw that he had three bullet wounds, which were about seven to ten days old. Had he made the tracks found with those of the poached pair? One of his wounds was in the right shoulder, one was in his skull above the frontal sinus, and the third consisted of an entry and exit wound below the right ear near the angle of his lower jaw. We cleaned the wounds, flushed them with antibiotic preparations, and injected the rhino with intramuscular antibiotics. "The Little Guy," as we initially named him, traveled well by truck to Serowe and was released into his own boma the next morning.

The young bull's boma was between those of the old bull on one side and the cow and calf on the other. The Little Guy had difficulty settling in. He was the most aggressive of the animals, often charging the shade-cloth-covered walls of the wooden bomas when caretakers approached. He spent a fair amount of time appearing to seek social interaction with the cow and calf, rubbing up against the fence separating the two bomas and calling to them in high-pitched vocalizations classified as "whining" and "squeaking." He sounded almost guinea pig–like, but with a slower cadence.

Biologists have differentiated rhino vocalizations. The whining noise The Little Guy made was considered a juvenile begging call; the squeaking, a juvenile distress call. Given his behavior, his age, and the spoor (tracks) found near his capture site, it seemed quite certain that the cow and calf killed just before the capture operation were indeed the mother and younger sibling of this little bull. The Little Guy was more than a little lonely.

Not only did he feel alone, but he also wouldn't eat. Post-capture inappetence is a frequent problem that can be life-threatening in free-ranging white rhinos placed into captivity. Some animals, especially older bulls, will not eat for the first week or ten days (or longer) postcapture. As a result, rhino bomas are generally situated in the same areas where the rhinos are being captured. Grasses can then be cut at the capture sites and offered to newly confined animals. If a rhino refuses this local food and continues its hunger strike, it can be released from the boma back into the park without any further transport. But, for security reasons, our rhino sanctuary had to be located far from the capture site. Release into the land adjacent to the sanctuary, part of the eventual plan, was not an option at the time—money was still being raised to build the necessary perimeter fence.

The calf was the first to eat postcapture, having suckled within twenty-four hours. Its mother started eating on day four, and the adult bull two days later. But by day ten, The Little Guy had taken only a few bites of grass. His behavior surprised us, as it's usually the older bulls that refuse to eat. We offered the young bull grasses cut at the capture site, a variety of fresh fruits, and even fresher local grasses. He ignored them all. We even tried coating some of the grass with molasses, a tactic I'd employed successfully in a zoo setting—but to no avail. The rhino was drinking water, he appeared bright and alert, but he just wouldn't eat. We had to do something to get him to take in sustenance.

First, I needed to determine the cause of the little bull's

anorexia. Was this the "classic" confinement-related response?
Given his subadult age and the good appetite of the adult
male, we thought not. Could his wounds be causing a diminished appetite? There was no way to assess his injuries at this
point without further anesthesia, and I was not ready to risk
additional postanesthesia inappetence or to further disturb
him or the other animals by darting him and working inside
the boma. Besides, The Little Guy was not showing other
overt signs of being a sick animal: no lethargy, no depression.
He was plenty active, appearing to be seeking rhino-to-rhino
interaction. We decided to give the little bull the social contact he seemed to want.

There were two choices: put him with the mother and
calf or with the adult bull. Both were risky options. If we put
the young bull with the family pair, we could upset the cow,
potentially interfering with her care of the calf. There was
also the danger that The Little Guy would injure the calf. On
the other hand, if we put the two bulls together, we ran the
risk of extreme injury to the younger bull. Wild-caught
rhinos from different social groups and different ages/size
classes tend not to get along when put together in tight
spaces.

Yet the two bulls could now see each other (since the rhinos had ripped down all of the shade-cloth that had been
serving as a visual barrier between bomas), and the big bull
did not seem disturbed by The Little Guy's presence. We decided the lesser risk was to remove the barrier between the
two bulls—and to be prepared to separate them again if all
did not go well.

Twelve days postcapture, the gate between the two males

was removed. Nothing happened at first. We watched nervously for an hour. Finally, the young bull crossed over to his senior's boma. I held my breath. Initially, he was escorted back out by the big bull ("Ol' Boss" is what we were calling him at this point). But, much to our joy and relief, there was no aggression. The Little Guy headed right back into the older bull's boma and followed him around constantly. And the old bull let him.

The Little Guy had now all but stopped charging the fence, a clear departure from his previously agitated behavior. And when Ol' Boss went to eat, The Little Guy ate with him! Over the course of the day, the older bull would occasionally horn his new boma-mate in the axilla (armpit), but this seemed more a reminder to let elders eat or drink first than a serious attempt to dominate him. Eventually, Ol' Boss even let The Little Guy lie next to him when they rested.

On the second and third days of the housing experiment, days thirteen and fourteen postcapture, the young bull continued to eat small amounts. He even defecated on day fourteen. (We veterinarians love the arrival of a long-awaited bowel movement!) The Little Guy seemed content for those three days. And then came day fifteen: the little bull appeared weak and depressed. Given how well he'd responded to companionship, I now considered bullet-related infection to be at the root of his symptoms. He was now refusing to eat again.

When the rhino first refused to eat, we'd considered additional antibiotic therapy. But an animal of his size would need a large-volume dart delivered periodically into thigh or neck muscle, something that very much disturbs the patient on the receiving end. We also didn't want to disrupt his acclimation period in the boma. Plus, antibiotics can induce their own gastrointestinal disturbances, and I had not wanted to risk adding to the little bull's as-yet-unexplained anorexia when he looked so bright and alert otherwise.

Whether your patient is a wild animal or a pet—or even a person—every treatment option comes with an implicit cost-benefit analysis. This calculation is especially tricky in a case like this where getting even basic laboratory or other diagnostic work done easily and safely was impossible. We had no clinic, no rhino-handling facilities, just our experience and intuition. Now that the young bull clearly appeared ill, the risk of upsetting him was less than the risk of losing him to infection. He was started on a broad-spectrum antibiotic by dart. We also began supplementing his drinking water with dextrose, sucrose, and B-complex vitamin syrup.

On the following day, I added electrolytes to The Little Guy's water and darted him again with antibiotic. It was now seventeen days postcapture, and the little bull was doing poorly. We had been observing him around the clock, and had not seen him eat anything. I made the decision, in consultation with the on-site board members of the Khama Rhino Sanctuary, to immobilize him that day for more intensive care.

I administered a low dose of etorphine hydrochloride to anesthetize The Little Guy. He responded quickly to the narcotic. While constantly monitoring the rhino's heart rate, respiratory rate, and blood oxygenation (by pulse oximetry), I gave him oxygen intranasally as an extra precaution, given his debilitated condition. A flexible tube passed into his stomach allowed for the administration of a calorically dense multisource carbohydrate/amino acid/vegetable oil/vitamin/ electrolyte liquid mixture. I also administered intravenous fluids to treat dehydration, more antibiotics, and an injection of vitamins and minerals. When anesthesia was reversed with an injection of the antidote, the little bull immediately sat up, shook his head, and walked away.

On day eighteen postcapture, on March 5, 1993, at five PM local time, Botswana's bravest rhino died. I was devastated, perhaps more so by this loss than by the loss of any other patient I'd ever had. Fifteen years later, I still feel a bleak numbness when I think about seeing him dead in the boma. Saving him had been a moral imperative. His death seemed like an affirmation that all was not well with the world—that the bad guys had won.

I thought back to my small animal internship days and to my days as a zoo veterinarian as well. The truth is, people cause much of the suffering we deal with as veterinarians. Whether it's cats hit by cars, or dogs that have eaten rat poison, or seals that have swallowed the coins zoo visitors carelessly throw into their pools, the veterinarian constantly finds him- or herself trying to pick up the pieces, figuratively and literally, because of thoughtless, selfish, cruel, or stupid human acts. This little rhino with bullet wounds was no different. He was another animal who had been perfectly healthy the moment before he ran into a member of our species, one who happened to have a gun.

Emotionally drained, I performed the necropsy in the boma where The Little Guy had spent his last days. I found that the bullet that had entered the right shoulder prior to capture had passed all the way through the chest and abdomen, where it had caused further damage, leading to diffuse infection and his death. From the start, I had hoped that those bullet wounds did not go as deep as it was now obvious they had. The 7.62mm–caliber round, which I found in the rhino's abdomen, came from the type of semiautomatic weapon regional rhino poachers were famous for.

This was no zoo or university setting—I had no X-rays or MRIs and even had to scramble to find some of the drugs we'd needed. But I knew I had done my absolute best in this remote setting. My veterinary colleagues in the region were astounded that a wildlife vet kept an emergency oxygen tank and equipment like endotracheal tubes on hand, never mind a portable blood oxygen monitor. But this was still ultimately bush medicine, and doing my best had meant making do with locally available materials, just as I'd envisioned years earlier.

Everyone at the sanctuary was saddened by the loss of The Little Guy. We had rooted for him day and night and come to know him. He had tried so hard to make it. But we took great solace in the fact that he hadn't died alone. Instead of following the rules laid out in capture books and lore, we'd read the rhino's desires and provided him with the companionship he craved. I believe his last days were made more bearable because we'd taken a calculated risk to let him be with Ol' Boss. I could only guess that Ol' Boss must have been wondering what had happened to his little gray shadow.

Although we'd managed to capture and transport him to a safe place, and had helped him acclimate to captivity with an unorthodox intervention, the poachers who were decimating his kind got him in the end. At least they did not get his small horn. Posthumously, we renamed him Lerumo, "bullet" in the local Setswana language. I felt that this name fit him, and the sad situation, best.

Overall, the 1993 rhino translocation project was a pioneering success for the DWNP in terms of accomplishments and the staff training it provided—success that would not have been possible without our Natal Parks Board colleagues. The Khama Rhino Sanctuary continues its conservation and education mission. An additional male was captured in 1994, calves have been born, and South Africa has donated several more rhinos to Botswana, some of which are back in the wild, this time under much more intensive protection than in the past. I think of them as Lerumo's legacy.

ABOUT THE AUTHOR

Steven A. Osofsky is a wildlife veterinarian with a long-standing focus on international conservation. His first experience in Africa was as a Harvard University Traveling Fellow in 1984. He attended veterinary school at Cornell University, receiving his doctor of veterinary medicine degree in 1989. Dr. Osofsky went to Botswana in 1991 to serve as the government of Botswana's first Wildlife Veterinary Officer, a post he left in 1994. He has also worked as a clinical zoological veterinarian, as an American Association for the Advancement of Science fellow and biodiversity specialist for the US Agency for International Development, and as director of field support for the World Wildlife Fund's (WWF-US) Species Conservation Program. The author of more than thirty scientific papers and book chapters, he is currently senior policy advisor for wildlife health for the Wildlife Conservation Society (WCS), with a focus on the wildlife/domestic animal/human health interface. He and his veterinarian wife, Dr. Karen J. Hirsch, have two young children who so far seem to like animals.

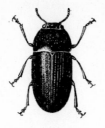

The Bugs Have Bugs?

by Maryanne Tocidlowski, DVM

I had mixed emotions when a supervisor from the children's zoo—part of the Houston Zoo, where I worked as staff veterinarian—called to say that their collection of dung beetles had red spots on them. Could I come take a look? There were seven beetles, from the *Canthon* genus; they'd been collected locally in Texas. I thought to myself, *I don't do bugs; I don't know anything about insects. I guess I could go look at them at least; maybe I can do something, but what?*

Like most budding veterinarians, I had a small collection of my own pets as a child, I loved science and animals—at least, most of them—and if I found an injured or sick wild creature, I'd try to take care of it. But insects and spiders had never interested me. I don't like being surprised by bugs landing on my shoulder or getting caught in my hair. I'm actually a little afraid of them. At best, they are nice to look at—through glass.

The beetles needed to be examined, however, and it was in my job description to pay them a visit. I began by doing some research on my soon-to-be patients. The Internet (in 2000) had no information about the medical management of dung beetles, nor any reference to beetles with red spots, but I did learn that dung beetles are very interesting creatures. Sometimes called "tumblebugs," most species are between 1 and 1½ inches long; the color of their carapace, or body, ranges from dull to shiny black. Considered environmentally beneficial and medically harmless, these beetles recycle animal feces. On a Texas ranch, they can recycle up to 80 percent of the cattle manure in a pasture, improving soil nutrient levels and structure, and supporting forage growth for the cattle to eat.

Different species of dung beetle found in other parts of the world play a similar role, ensuring a healthy environment for animals as varied as gazelles, rhinos, and elephants. Adult beetles use the liquid portion of manure for nourishment, sort of a dung Slurpee (sorry, but that's the image this fact created in my mind). Then they work in male-female pairs to roll a ball of dung away from the manure pile, and the female lays an egg in the middle of the ball. They bury it in a deep burrow. The egg develops into a larva, which then eats its way out of the dung ball and to the surface, to start the life cycle all over again.

I also got a bit distracted reading about ancient Egypt. The dung beetle was once considered sacred by the Egyptians. The beetle's behavior of rolling a huge dung ball during the day, disappearing into a hole at night, and starting again the next day symbolized renewal and a connection to the god of the rising sun. There was also a belief that all dung beetles were male, reproducing themselves out of nothing by depositing sperm into the dung ball. Had bugs been my hobby growing up, maybe I would have known all of this.

After learning what I could, I met the children's zoo supervisor to go look at the beetles. On our way, I kept thinking—hoping—that maybe we'd find nothing wrong with them. But I soon saw that all seven dung beetles actually did have red spots and that the spots moved. They appeared to be some type of millimeter-size red insect riding around on their backs. My best guess was a mite.

At that point, I realized that the difference between a beetle and a mite confused me. Both are in the kingdom Animalia and phylum Arthropoda, which makes them generically "bugs." They diverge from there. Mites belong to the class Arachnida, same as spiders and ticks, and dung beetles belong to the class Insecta, along with wasps, ants, grasshoppers, butterflies, other types of beetles, and—just to confuse the issue—a particular type of insect called a "true bug." So both were bugs: the mites were arachnids and the beetles were insects.

I had plenty of questions about this case. I'd never had to work on a bug infested with bugs. Were the red bugs harmful to the beetles, or were they symbiotic bugs just hitching a ride? Would they go away on their own? Where had they come from? How would I handle these animals if I needed to?

I remembered seeing mites on other types of animals, like chiggers that bite humans and cause a rash. I'd seen little red mites on the bodies of birds and reptiles; these are harmful to the animal because they bite and suck blood, potentially causing anemia, or passing bacteria or viruses to their hosts. But even if these beetle hitchhikers were similar to those seen on humans, birds, or reptiles, the treatment would have to be completely different. For animals infested with mites, we use commercially available insecticides—carefully. A more appropriate name for such chemicals might be "bugicides." In this case, they would undoubtedly kill my patients as well as their red spots.

I asked more questions about the history of the zoo's beetles and the red mites: were the dung beetles behaving, eating, and moving around normally? The responses were not helpful: "We're not sure" and "They don't seem to be eating as much as before." Given the number of red mites observed on each beetle, I decided reluctantly that this was a problem that needed taking care of. The supervisor and I discussed the situation and came up with a plan—several plans, actually.

First, we would try to change their environment. The mulch substrate for the beetles could be the source of the infestation; maybe the red mites normally live in this soil. So we brought in fresh dirt, hoping the hitchhikers would prefer it to the beetles. After a few days, we saw no difference. The beetles still had red spots, mostly congregated around the midbody, near what I would call the neck region. Next we tried freezing the soil for several days before using it. Maybe this step would kill the mites already in the substrate and reduce the numbers on the beetles. But when we placed the beetles and their red friends on the thawed-out soil, the hitchhikers still did not disappear.

Okay, on to the next step.

The conservative approach had failed. I would need to manually remove the red mites from the beetles. But this strategy presented yet another set of questions: How could I get the mites off without harming my patients or myself? If I put the dung beetles in an anesthetic chamber to anesthetize them, then removed them to work on them, would they stay asleep long enough? If I dispensed with the chamber, was there any way I could use anesthetic gas on the beetles without putting myself to sleep as well?

Since I couldn't think of a way to keep the beetles under anesthesia long enough to work on them, that option was out. I would have to contain my fear of bugs and somehow immobilize the beetles myself while I picked off the red mites.

The removal operation was scheduled for one quiet afternoon, and the dung beetles were brought up to the clinic. I didn't know how they'd react to the stress of my handling and fussing over them, so we split the beetle collection in two. One group of three would go back to the children's zoo exhibit to be the "control group"; the four others would be the "experimental manual removal group."

The day before, I'd asked my technicians to sterilize some dirt so that it was free of all possible contamination. Even more surely than freezing, the sterilization process would kill any bacteria, fungi, or bugs that might be lingering in the soil. Once they were cleared of the red bugs, the beetles would be kept in the sterilized dirt in a clean cage at the clinic for monitoring. I'm pretty sure this was the one and only time we purposefully put dirt into our clean sterilizing unit.

Now the fun part began. What should I use to restrain these little buggers? Even if the beetles could tolerate the stress of hands-on handling, I feared my instruments or clumsiness might damage them beyond repair. We might need to modify my technique as we proceeded, depending on the results, good or bad. The supervisor and staff understood the risks. Ready to proceed, I chose a pair of large blunt-tipped forceps (surgical tweezers, about six inches long, with rounded tips) to handle the beetles, allowing me to control the pressure on the body. I chose a pair of small delicate forceps about four inches long, with pointy tips, to remove the red mites from the beetles. I set a shallow plate in front of me to serve as a catch pan in case the dung beetle fell from my grasp, or in case one of us needed a break.

The first procedure on any animal is always a learning experience. I grabbed the first beetle and it jumped! Startled, I gasped, and half rose from my chair. Everyone in the room laughed, including me, even while I thought, *Please don't jump or fly onto me.* Luckily, the first beetle didn't go far; it jumped just enough to let me know it wasn't happy with my touching it. At least it didn't fly. These beetles have large wings that enable them to move from dung pile to dung pile in the wild. (My worst fear was of a beetle flying around my treatment room, pursued by people running after it with nets.)

The next time I grabbed the beetle, I held it firmly but gently—and held my breath at the same time. Once the beetle realized I wasn't letting go, it stopped struggling, played dead, and behaved like an ideal patient throughout the rest of the procedure. I had to scout around on its small black body, peering in all the cracks and crevices for red bugs. It took about a quarter of an hour to remove all the mites.

Each of the four beetles I treated that first day handled the procedure like a champ. They were placed in the cage with the sterilized soil and kept at the clinic for a week. All survived without any obvious signs of trauma. No red mites were detected on the beetles during the observation period. A week later, the three beetles of the control group back at the children's zoo were brought to the clinic to undergo the same procedure. Again, all went well, and we put them in the sterile-environment cage with their friends from the first group.

After the keepers had disinfected their habitat cage, we returned the group of seven beetles to their original exhibit, along with a fresh batch of sterile soil. They were home again. I visited them daily for a week. So far, so good: they were behaving normally, without freeloading bugs. But a month later, I got a report that the red mites were back, although in far fewer numbers. We decided to leave them alone and just be vigilant, since the beetles appeared healthy. If the situation changed, I would intervene again.

I never found out for sure what those little red bugs were, though it's likely that they were parasitic mites. I suppose we could have sent them to a special lab for identification, but I doubt that would have changed the outcome. Generally, the mites didn't seem to be doing any harm to the beetles. Plus, my attempted treatment hadn't worked, and I doubt I would have tried anything more invasive. Any kind of chemical just seemed too dangerous for the patient.

After all the hours I spent on this case, I still knew very little about insect medicine. Did the mites make the beetles feel itchy, lethargic, or thirsty? I have no idea, and doubt I ever will.

I'm happy to say that I haven't been asked to examine or treat any of our other bugs—though that may just be a matter of time. On the other hand, the thought of spending a quiet afternoon in the clinic picking mites off dung beetles no longer bugs me.

ABOUT THE AUTHOR

Maryanne Tocidlowski was raised in New York State and decided to become a vet at the age of ten. She graduated from Daemen College in Buffalo, New York, as a medical technologist, and then worked in a human hospital hematology laboratory for six years before attending veterinary technician school. Dr. Tocidlowski graduated with an associate's degree in animal health technology and was then accepted to Purdue University's College of Veterinary Medicine. After her graduation in 1993, she did a one-year small animal internship at the New Haven Central Animal Hospital in Connecticut; next came a three-year residency in zoological medicine at North Carolina State University and the North Carolina Zoological Park. Dr. Tocidlowski joined the staff of the Houston Zoo in 1997 as an associate veterinarian, and became a diplomate of the American College of Zoological Medicine in 1998.

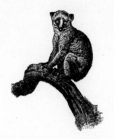

Death of a Lemur:
An Unsolved Mystery

by Amy Rae Gandolf, DVM

I stiffened with anxious tension as I opened my e-mail to read the final pathology report on Brass, the red-ruffed lemur. I hoped for confirmation of the immune disease I'd suspected, or at least some sort of clue to the cause of the lemur's fatal illness. But as I scanned the report, anticipation gave way to disappointment and my questions remained unanswered. I sighed and slumped in my chair, studying the screen to review the details I'd hurried through on the first read. No, I hadn't missed anything. I sat back, replaying the case in my mind in a last-ditch search for answers to the bizarre illness.

I couldn't help feeling as if I'd failed Brass. Part of my reaction was personal. This case hit a little too close to home. I'd wanted to find an answer in the report not only to satisfy myself but also to share it with my mom. Coincidentally, she too had been suffering from strange chronic ailments. The past few months, we'd talked over the phone every week or two about both her case and the lemur's. Where they overlapped, we'd compared clues as we tried to solve the mysteries.

Lemurs are primitive tree-dwelling primates with long, furry tails. They are distinct from monkeys and found only in Madagascar. Most photographs show the ring-tailed species; they tend to gather in photogenic groups that display their brilliant raccoonlike faces, white bellies, and striking black-and-white striped tails.

Brass was a red-ruffed lemur, equally attractive and curious. The red-ruffs are orange-red with black hands and faces. Their bodies are more compact and their coats fluffier than those of the ring-tails. With their unhurried gait, boundless curiosity, fuzzy bodies, and little hands, they sometimes look like creatures straight out of Dr. Seuss.

Early in my position as associate veterinarian at the Pittsburgh Zoo, the red-ruffs in the collection became favorites. Two of them had minor medical issues, and they all required routine health checks, so I got to know the group fairly quickly. I developed a great fondness for them and always enjoyed an excuse to visit. For a closer look at Brass or one of the others, I'd walk into their enclosure with their keeper and some food treats. I'd hold out a grape and await the inevitable eager response—inquisitive big brown eyes and open hands. While my attention was fixed on one lemur, I often felt another sneaking up behind me to toy curiously with my keys or radio. The more time I spent with the lemurs, the more endearing they became.

Brass's medical problems surfaced in July 2005, with his regularly scheduled health exam. As with most zoo animals, the exam required anesthesia. On that particular day, we examined him and Copper, the other male in the group. The morning went smoothly and according to plan, a team effort among myself; the zoo's head veterinarian, Dr. Cindy Stadler; our technician, Libby; and Karen, the lead primate keeper. A writer and photographer from a local newspaper viewed Brass's exam as part of an ongoing zoo storyline they'd been developing.

Each exam took about an hour, including a full physical, radiographs, teeth cleaning, blood and stool collection for testing, and a tuberculosis (TB) skin test, a routine screening test in primates. To check for TB, we inject a tenth of a milliliter of a special reagent, tuberculin, in the upper eyelid and watch for swelling over the next few days. This test is used in people too, but the injection is given in the forearm. A human will readily extend an arm so the nurse can read the test, but primates aren't usually that cooperative. Instead, we use the eyelid so that any resultant swelling can be easily seen from a short distance.

Brass was in great condition and received a clean bill of health. His laboratory results would return the following week and show no cause for concern, although his red blood cells were at the low end of the normal range. When Brass was checked the day after his exam, however, his eyelid TB test site was swollen. Over the next two days, the swelling increased to include both eyes and his muzzle. We interpreted this response as a nonspecific TB test reaction rather than a true positive, since positive tests have distinct features that we didn't see in Brass, including a very red and inflamed eyelid.

We regarded Brass's strange facial swelling as a nonspecific reaction to something in the tuberculin. Or he could have been exposed to any number of TB-like organisms found naturally in the environment that can cause a false positive test. We made plans to reanesthetize Brass in a few weeks for follow-up testing to prove he didn't have TB.

Meanwhile, a nice article about Brass's checkup came out in the paper, with a picture of Karen holding him as he recovered from anesthesia. I clipped it and sent it to my mom, who didn't remember what a lemur was until she saw the picture. An avid amateur photographer, she'd planned to come down from Connecticut to visit me at the zoo for a behind-the-scenes tour—a chance to photograph the animals up close. Unfortunately, she had been experiencing some sort of progressive illness for the past several months, and wouldn't be able to make the trip until things turned around.

Most TB test reactions subside within a week. Brass's swelling lasted longer, though he seemed fine otherwise and had only minimal swelling after two weeks and several doses of ibuprofen and Benadryl. A few days before the follow-up exam was due, I was surprised and perplexed when Karen reported that the dramatic swelling had returned. That's when the case became unusual. We began to wonder if, among other possibilities, the condition could somehow be related to a particular problem known to affect red-ruffed lemurs, called proliferative bone disease.

We put Brass on prednisone (a stronger anti-inflammatory medicine than ibuprofen) and switched him to a different antihistamine. I sought advice from the official veterinary Species Survival Plan advisor for lemurs, Dr. Randy Junge. During our phone conversation, Dr. Junge said the only similar case in a lemur that he was aware of involved a less severe TB reaction that lasted a week before resolving on its own.

Since the strange swelling persisted, we decided it was time to reevaluate Brass under anesthesia in order to recheck his blood and obtain a tissue biopsy from his face. We also collected tracheal and stomach wash samples, a much more involved method of testing for TB. Those results came back negative several weeks later. Able to examine Brass closely with the anesthesia, we saw that he had some mild bleeding around his gums. We took radiographs of his skull; they were normal, as was the rest of his exam. We didn't find any sign of the bone disease that we'd wondered about. We collected blood in a special tube to check for bleeding disorders, but found no problems there, either.

Then, as Brass was waking up from the procedure, our technician, Libby, called from the microscope with alarming news: Brass had a dangerously low number of both red and white blood cells. Given that the lemur's behavior had been normal, this finding stunned everyone. It did explain, though, why Brass subsequently took an unusually long time to wake up from anesthesia.

I left a message that afternoon for Dr. Guillermo Couto, a renowned veterinary hematologist and oncologist, and coincidentally one of my professors in veterinary school. He was someone whose opinion I valued greatly. I went through the case with him the next morning, and faxed him the lemur's laboratory results. After reviewing the information, he said

Brass was not making new blood cells to nearly the degree he should be. We narrowed the likely causes to cancer, various possible infections, or an immune-mediated disease. The prognosis, he concluded, could be anywhere from treatable to catastrophic.

We started Brass on a strong antibiotic, continued his prednisone, and planned a bone marrow biopsy to narrow the list of possible diagnoses, or differentials, further. Because immature white and red blood cells are found in the bone marrow, the biopsy would show Dr. Couto which cells were involved in the lemur's disease. Blood cell abnormalities fall into only so many categories, regardless of the species, so the biopsy would help categorize Brass's illness. If Dr. Couto couldn't make a definitive diagnosis from the biopsy, he could at least suggest the two or three most likely possibilities.

Though the lemur now showed some signs of fatigue, he appeared normal otherwise. The bone marrow procedure went well, but we found a new swelling between Brass's rear legs during the exam. We sent one biopsy each to the local pediatric hospital, to Dr. Couto, and to a pathologist specializing in zoo animals. Two days later, the results brought good news, and all three labs concurred. We were able to rule out cancer. Even though Brass's blood cell counts were still well below normal, the sample showed that his bone marrow was functioning normally, trying to replace the cells at a rapid rate.

With these results, we'd narrowed our differentials to two broad disease categories: chronic infection and immune-mediated disease. Like humans, animals can develop autoimmune disease that causes their immune systems to recognize their own blood cells as foreign, destroying them as they are produced from the bone marrow. Often it's not known what triggers this abnormal immune response.

That's when I started to think almost daily about my mom and her own puzzling illness. Wishing I could help her more, I'd tried to offer encouragement and suggestions over the phone as her undiagnosed symptoms became more dramatic. Until a few weeks ago, there'd been no explanation for why she'd been able to kayak and take photographs two years ago but now could hardly hold up a camera, never mind paddle across a lake. After a year of increasing frustration and despair, the problem had recently become severe enough to cause abnormalities in her blood tests. She was finally diagnosed with polymyositis, an immune disease in which the muscle cells, including the diaphragm, are damaged by the body—as if they are foreign.

As I researched articles and talked to my mom, I began to see similarities between her condition and the lemur's. For instance, they were both on prednisone to keep an undesirable immune system response at bay. As Brass had ups and downs, I asked a lot about her medication doses and how they affected her, as well as about her other treatments and symptoms. In the past, we'd never talked much about the details of my job, but now we often spoke about the lemur.

I was so used to comparing and contrasting conditions in all sorts of species, including humans, it didn't occur to me that my mom might be offended by my "comparing her to a monkey" until she commented on it. (I tried to explain that lemurs aren't actually monkeys, but I guess that wasn't the point.) She quickly got over that and became interested in the case. As she searched the Web about her own condition, she relayed tidbits and articles that she thought might apply to Brass. As I researched the lemur's condition, I did the same for her.

The week after his bone marrow biopsy, Brass looked brighter and less swollen than he had in two months. I was encouraged, thinking that whether the problem was a subsiding infection or an abnormal immune response, he was finally headed in the right direction. But the respite was short-lived. A week later, he was badly swollen once again. The pathologist felt that results of his initial facial biopsy in conjunction with those of his bone marrow supported the diagnosis of immune-mediated blood cell disease—with a poor prognosis. Dr. Couto agreed but thought that remission might still be a possibility.

Soon the struggle to control Brass's immune system became more difficult. We tried to strike a balance: dial down the response attacking his own cells, but not so far that he could no longer fight off ordinary bacteria and other infections. Karen sadly reported that Brass was finally beginning to look the way his lab results said he should. He began to suffer from various new problems related to his abnormal immune system. We tried to tackle new infections with strong antibiotics and antifungal medicines.

Brass submitted to being captured in a towel once a week so we could monitor his condition and blood work. Over the next two months, his blood counts and swellings fluctuated. We suspected his immune disease had become refractory—that is, it would no longer respond to our treatments. The lemur felt better on some days than others, putting his care-givers on an emotional roller coaster.

I tried to keep my own emotions suppressed. I think every veterinarian struggles with this at times. We get attached to our patients, but if we start worrying too much about the outcome, it's hard to stay focused on the diagnosis and treat-ment. So I try to strike a balance in my own mind, and create some degree of emotional distance. In some cases it's eas-ier said than done, especially with chronically ill animals whom we inevitably get to know well. But I couldn't deny my bond with this charming and forgiving little lemur. I wanted so much to find the answer, and I held on to hope for his recovery.

Meanwhile my mom began to sound more hopeful over the phone. She wasn't feeling any better, but she had seen a new specialist and was going to start an intravenous im-munoglobulin treatment regimen we'd considered for the lemur. As with Brass, the other drugs she was taking weren't helping nearly enough and were causing her many new prob-lems. When I'd called Dr. Couto to ask his opinion about the possibility of immunoglobulin treatment, he wasn't very en-couraging. I later discovered that at ten thousand dollars per treatment for a human, this very slim possibility for a cure could not have been an option for the lemur. I was thankful for my mom's health insurance, and hoped this treatment would give her the help she needed.

Brass grew quite accustomed to our visits. In the past, he'd always been a bit shy, more timid than the other lemurs. Now he seemed to enjoy an occasional scratch on the back. Every time I looked at him, I searched for something I'd missed.

When I scratched his back, I'd feel his vertebrae and gauge his body condition; I'd gradually move my hands toward his head and touch his swollen face, hoping for fresh inspiration.

But the weeks slipped by, and instead of finding answers, I was increasingly forced to face defeat. Karen felt that Brass was beginning to go downhill quickly. We found him curled up near the warmth of the heat lamp more frequently, and what appeared to be a sprained pinky finger escalated into a hand so swollen that his skin began to split. Brass also began losing weight, despite special food supplements.

As I watched Brass one day, Karen and I talked about his degree of suffering and his increasingly poor prognosis. Without mentioning the word "euthanasia," I knew we felt the same way. We hated to give up hope, but we didn't want Brass to continue suffering from something he would not overcome. The zoo's head vet, Cindy, and I discussed the matter with our technicians; everyone agreed, as did the other primate keepers, the curator, and the zoo director. It was a Friday. We decided that if Brass did not show improvement from our latest treatments by the following week, we wouldn't let him suffer any longer.

When I talked to my mom that weekend, I hated telling her the news. She expressed concern, knowing how much I'd wanted to save Brass. She'd been pulling for him too, and I wondered if it bothered her to find me admitting defeat against problems that were vaguely similar to her own.

Monday, my day off, I got a message from Cindy saying that Brass had really deteriorated and they'd decided to euthanize him. Although I'd hoped to be there, I didn't want him to suffer and was glad they were going to help him in the only way left to them.

Once the battle was over, all I could hope for was some sort of answer from the examination of his body so that we could keep this from happening to another lemur. We sent many samples to the pathologist for tests and microscopic evaluation—and waited. Two weeks later, I received the report I mentioned earlier: nothing.

Before I began writing Brass's story, I retrieved his medical chart, intending to refer to it to recall time frames and treatments more accurately. Instead, I found myself wrapped up in the case all over again, reviewing clinical entries and lab reports from start to finish, and trying once more to find something I'd missed. His case affected me on a personal level more than most. This gentle lemur suffered from a complex disease that we never figured out. The harsh reality is that we don't always find the answer in zoo medicine—or in human medicine.

As for my mom, her story is thankfully taking a different turn. Six months after starting immunoglobulin therapy, she began to notice subtle improvements. A year after that, still on the monthly immunoglobulin treatments, she was finally well enough to visit me and the Pittsburgh Zoo. Copper and the other lemurs were some of her first photographic subjects in over two years.

I will always wonder about what happened to Brass and why, and I will always wonder if a different course of treatment could have changed the outcome. When I stop wondering, I suppose that's when I'll stop growing as a veterinarian.

ABOUT THE AUTHOR

Originally from East Haddam, Connecticut, Amy Rae Gandolf developed a passion for wildlife as a child, an interest she pursued during veterinary school at Ohio State University. She gained field experience through volunteer work with wildlife conservation and rehabilitation organizations from Ohio to Guatemala to Thailand—experience that was strengthened by further training in a veterinary residency at the Wilds, a wildlife conservation center in Ohio. Following her residency, Dr. Gandolf worked as an associate veterinarian at the Pittsburgh Zoo and PPG Aquarium. In addition to working with species of various shapes and sizes in clinical practice, Dr. Gandolf has been involved in a number of research projects: issues of environmental toxicants affecting wildlife in both the US and Uganda, brown bear health in Sweden, and pharmacokinetic studies with zoo animals. Her ardor for free-ranging wildlife, research, and travel continues to inspire her efforts to aid in the ongoing development and improvement of wildlife management.

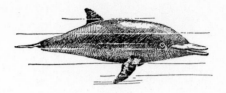

Baker D

by Marty Haulena, DVM, MSc

What's best for a stranded bottlenose dolphin? Why do they end up on the beach in the first place? How can we improve their chances of survival when we first rescue them? And how do we know where and how to release them if they survive their initial rehabilitation? These questions, along with our best efforts to answer them, occupied a great many discussions among The Marine Mammal Center staff and volunteers in Sausalito, California.

Most stranded cetaceans (dolphins, porpoises, and whales) die in the first twenty-four to forty-eight hours after rescue. The cause of death is often a chain of problems that begin the moment the animal finds itself on the beach. No longer suspended in water, it suffers from the weight of its own body. Not only does a stranded dolphin have difficulty breathing, its skin and muscles bruise quickly from pressure on the hard ground.

Biochemically, the animal begins to suffer too. A series of chemical changes are triggered by the dolphin's stress reaction to being out of water in a foreign environment. If it could, the dolphin would struggle or flee—the fight-or-flight reaction that is universal among mammals in stressful situations, fueled by the chemical epinephrine, or adrenaline. Unable to move, the dolphin's epinephrine builds to an excessively high level, which then damages the muscles further. Since the heart is one of the largest muscles in the body, the chemical becomes life-threatening rather than lifesaving.

Recent advances in our understanding of the physiological changes going on inside a stranded dolphin have helped our rescue efforts at the Center, and we've improved our success rate over the last decade or so. By the time Baker D arrived, in September 2004, we had better techniques for transport, stabilization, diagnostic procedures, and therapy. But supporting a stranded animal all the way back to a successful release into the wild was still a very rare event.

We put all of our knowledge to work when this young male dolphin came in. Lifeguards had found him stranded on Baker D Beach, and named him accordingly. They carried him on a stretcher to the nearest parking lot, where I first met this special dolphin. Already weak and unable to move, Baker D watched wide-eyed as we scrambled around him. I wondered what he thought of these noisy, unfamiliar humans poking and prodding him. A young male, he was alert and had relatively few wounds despite the time he'd spent on dry land. We knew his chances of survival were pretty good, all things considered. But the helpless dolphin, completely out of his element, had no idea what would happen next.

People often try to help stranded dolphins by pushing them back into the water, only to have them re-strand and eventually die. They don't understand that the stress of stranding has created a host of new problems that threaten its survival, in or out of the water. At least Baker D would escape that fate. We would carefully stabilize him; if he made it, we would begin the long process of rehabilitation. Though I knew the odds were probably against us, I felt that Baker D was a strong candidate for eventual release. Whatever the outcome, we would learn something from the case.

We started supportive therapy right away, first by injecting Baker D with a general sedative. We placed a catheter into a vein in his tail fluke so we could give him a variety of IV drugs, including more sedative (Valium), corticosteroids, antibiotics, and propranolol, a drug that would lower the dolphin's heart rate and protect the heart tissue. Then we hooked up a rehydration fluid drip for his transport to The Marine Mammal Center, a relatively short thirty-minute drive.

Staff had readied a soft-sided pool for Baker D, twenty-four feet in diameter and three and a half feet deep. With our lab technicians prepared to analyze the samples, we took blood for diagnostic and research purposes, including DNA testing, weighed him, and carefully moved him to the pool in a stretcher.

The moment we lowered the dolphin into the water, the real work began. Though the Center employs fifty people full-time, including three veterinarians, a group of about six hundred volunteers performs the bulk of the day-to-day hands-on animal care. These incredibly dedicated, caring people are essential to the critical care of stranded animals. Over the following weeks, they would nurse Baker D.

Initially, Baker D could neither swim nor support himself in the water. So our volunteers fashioned a special sling made of floats and neoprene to help keep him afloat. Two people at a time stood in the water with the dolphin to guide him gently around the pool, preventing him from listing or sinking and injuring himself. On that first day, I also stayed with him for several hours, monitoring him and helping to develop a treatment plan with the rest of our excellent veterinary team. The next day, Baker D already appeared stronger. Within a week, he'd progressed significantly: his appetite had picked up and he'd adjusted to the people caring for him. He was still very weak, however. We had a long way to go.

For the next several weeks, our volunteers nursed the dolphin around the clock, often standing for hours in the cold water and misty coastal air. They fed him regularly, dosed him with medication, and kept detailed records for every minute of the day for several weeks. No one voiced a complaint, only concern for the special patient under their care. I can't say enough about the outstanding group of volunteers that is the heart and soul of The Marine Mammal Center. These are people who always try to do the right thing, who strive to improve themselves and the world around them, who simply care.

Gradually, Baker D became able to navigate the small pool on his own. As he continued to gain strength, we knew he'd need a deeper pool where he could get more exercise and conditioning for a potential release. We called the Long

Marine Laboratory at the University of California, Santa Cruz, whose staff graciously agreed to take Baker D and give him the space he needed. Another dedicated team of people took over his care. Though we'd all bonded to Baker D, this was a happy day. We were excited and proud to see a live animal leave the Center—on its way home.

Before long, Baker D was swimming in the big pool with speed and strength. It was time to plan for his release back to the wild. The first step was to review the conditions in which we'd found him initially.

Strandings often occur in areas where the coast slopes very gradually into shallow water, a geographic feature that makes echolocation, the system dolphins use to navigate, more difficult. Changes in sea level associated with global warming may play a role in the shallow-slope effect. Some believe noises associated with human activity, like boat engines, drilling, mining, and military operations, have a lot to do with strandings. Underwater noise may interfere with the dolphins' ability to navigate, damage their hearing, and even cause them to surface too quickly, resulting in "the bends." A group of dolphins can also strand when the dominant animal in a group becomes disoriented and leads the rest of the pod to disaster.

Another possibility in Baker D's case—and our greatest concern from a medical point of view—was the presence of an infectious disease we hadn't been able to diagnose. If a bacterial or viral infection had sickened him and caused him to strand, the same disease could be a danger to other dolphins when he was released. Perhaps toxins, whether from human or natural sources, had affected him.

However, we'd found no evidence of any infection. No

other dolphins had stranded at the same time; nor were there reports of any toxic spills during the period in question. Though there could have been other contributing factors, we believed that Baker D had simply made a mistake. A young, curious, and inexperienced male, maybe he'd ventured away from his pod hunting fish, unaware that he'd strayed too far. Maybe he'd gotten too close to shore and had been pummeled by waves onto the rocky beach. Or maybe he'd encountered an aggressive group of other dolphins or a potential predator that had chased him into the rough, shallow water.

Now we had what appeared to be a healthy dolphin living safely in a pool. How could we ensure we'd done our best to prepare him for a return to the ocean? Would he be able to find his pod?

We reviewed the established guidelines for releasing stranded dolphins. The animal should be in the best possible physical shape, free of diseases that might pose a danger to healthy wild animals; it should be fitted with a tracking device and released in the vicinity of members of the same species. We knew of a group of bottlenose dolphins that frequent Monterey Bay, coming close to shore at a certain stretch of beach almost every day. Our best guess was that Baker D belonged to this group of dolphins. So when, after two months of intense rehabilitation, we decided he was ready to go back to the wild, we made plans to release him in the bay.

On the day of his release, we fitted Baker D with both a VHF radio tag and a satellite-linked tag on his dorsal fin. These instruments are designed to detach themselves after approximately 250 to 300 days, their expected battery life. As soon as we spotted the group of wild dolphins, we headed out to sea by boat with Baker D safely aboard in a specially designed stretcher. About two hours later, we gently lowered the dolphin to the surface of the sea, positioning him to face the group of dolphins a hundred yards away. Once free of the stretcher, Baker D dove down, turned away from the other dolphins, swam under our boat, and disappeared under the water.

Our radio-tracking receiver picked up the sound from his VHF tag just once, as he porpoised out of the water—somewhere out of our sight. He swam away so fast that we never heard him again. Though his behavior was not what we'd expected, we were generally pleased with the outcome, proud to have completed such a rare but satisfying task. A job well done, or so we thought.

For the next few weeks, we received daily transmissions from Baker D's satellite-linked tag. Information about his location was transmitted to a satellite and then downloaded from the Internet to generate a map showing his precise post-release travels. Initially, Baker D seemed to be heading north toward San Francisco. But then he turned around and moved very quickly southward, reaching the Channel Islands off Santa Barbara. He made this trip in a little over a week, a distance of approximately 280 miles.

We couldn't help wondering why Baker D had moved so rapidly away from the area that had seemed natural for him, populated by other bottlenose dolphins. Could he be disoriented? Had we missed a disease, one of those that can cause permanent brain damage?

Once near the Channel Islands, Baker D's signals showed that he moved only small distances and stayed very close to land. Three weeks after his release, he was barely moving from one day to the next. On day seventy-six after release, the satellite-linked transmitter sent its last transmission. Not a good sign. We began to assume the worst.

At the Center we reviewed the pattern of satellite-location signals. The data seemed to indicate that Baker D had died. The relative lack of movement could mean that he'd been floating lifeless in the water. Thereafter, his body would have sunk to the ocean floor.

We were devastated. The volunteers and staff of The Marine Mammal Center and Long Marine Laboratory, the lifeguards and boat operators—we'd all worked so hard to give Baker D the best care, make the best medical decisions, and create the best possible scenario for his successful release. We wondered what we could have done differently. Maybe we should have tried to find a home for him in an aquarium. Perhaps we should have released him sooner or rehabilitated him longer. Were there other diagnostics we could have performed to find out what was wrong with him?

Two weeks after the last satellite signal, the Center's marine biologist, Denise Greig, and a number of people from Long Marine Laboratory, including the lead husbandry manager, Brett Long, decided it was worth chartering a research flight to have a look for Baker D's body. They hoped to gain some—any—information about what had happened to him. Even if the satellite-linked transmitter had failed, perhaps the VHF radio transmitter was still functional and would lead them to his body if it had washed up onshore.

I wasn't on the plane, but Denise and Brett told me all about it:

It was a stormy February day when the plane set forth on its grim mission. The clouds were heavy with rain, the rough weather buffeting the plane. As the day wore on, the plane flew intersecting search patterns. The crew was quiet, concentrating and listening, intent on picking up even the faintest signal from the radio transmitters in their headphones. Dusk was coming on and the fuel gauges showed the flight could not continue much longer.

Suddenly, the dark clouds parted and beams of golden sunshine shone down on the deep blue sea. Bright rays reflected off the peaks of the waves. A rainbow appeared in the late afternoon sky. The crew heard a faint "beep-beep-beep." It stopped and started again. Then it got louder and clearer before disappearing again. Illuminated by glowing sunlight, a large group of bottlenose dolphins—250 or more—suddenly sprang into view, moving fast. Right in the center, broadcasting his signal loud and clear every time he cleared the surface of the water, swam Baker D.

—

Months later, once the genetic analysis was completed (these special tests require a lot of time), we learned that Baker D didn't belong to the group of dolphins near Monterey Bay. He belonged to another well-known group of animals, the group that lives near the Channel Islands. Baker D was never lost. He knew all along where he was and where he belonged.

ABOUT THE AUTHOR

Martin Haulena graduated from the Ontario Veterinary College at the University of Guelph in 1993. He completed a clinical internship in aquatic animal medicine at Mystic Aquarium in 1996 and a master's degree in pathobiology from the University of Guelph in 1999. He served as the staff veterinarian at The Marine Mammal Center in Sausalito, California, for nine years, and is currently staff veterinarian at the Vancouver Aquarium in British Columbia. Dr. Haulena's special interests are in the medical management of aquatic animals, particularly marine mammals, with emphasis on innovative diagnostic methods such as MRIs, endoscopy, and ultrasonography, developing safe anesthetic protocols, and improving surgical techniques. Veterinary students from around the world study aquatic animal medicine each year under the direction of Dr. Haulena. His professional affiliations include the International Association for Aquatic Animal Medicine, the Wildlife Disease Association, and the American Association of Zoo Veterinarians.

V

CROSSOVER

Myriad anatomical and physiological differences exist among the animal groups, creating a special set of hurdles for the zoo vet. Even closely related species with the same condition may show different signs. The best medicine for a mammal may not work for a bird, reptile, amphibian, fish, or insect.

Fortunately, the basic principles of medicine do apply across species—human, domestic, and wild. Many vets who work with wild animals have also practiced on domestic animals at one time in their careers. Veterinary medicine for dogs, cats, horses, cows, and, to some extent, poultry is the basis of our formal education. From these species, we learn to extrapolate. Reptiles, for example, are evolutionarily closest to birds, so there is some crossover to chicken and turkey medicine. The more open-minded and flexible we are, the better we perform as zoo vets.

Kidney failure, for example, leads to a buildup of toxins in the blood that needs to be flushed out. The treatment is a combination of fluid therapy and modifications to the diet, plus antibiotics or other specific medicines, depending on the cause of the problem. In severe cases, dialysis can be used to keep the patient alive. When faced with a case of kidney failure, the zoo vet will typically review how this problem is diagnosed and treated in other, related species. The next step is to modify and fine-tune it to the animal's needs, with attention to the specifics of its species—physiology, anatomy, and disease susceptibility.

For example, an elephant with kidney failure becomes ill very rapidly. Such a patient requires vast quantities of fluids, over one hundred gallons a day, delivered intravenously and continuously if possible. How are these given? The ear veins work well if the elephant is trained to stand still for an intravenous catheter. Or the fluids can be given rectally with a garden hose, a technique also used for horses. Since acute bacterial infection is often the cause, strong antibiotics must be delivered quickly. Such a treatment plan requires a team of people and swift action.

By comparison, a desert iguana with kidney failure develops clinical signs much more gradually. It may show no signs of overt illness until just before death. Often its problem is not infection but rather a gradual buildup of precipitated protein by-products in the kidney. Because this species is evolved to conserve water, its cardiovascular system can handle only tiny amounts of intravenous fluids. An iguana in need of fluid therapy gets it just ounces at a time, once a day, under the skin. The subcutaneous delivery ensures slow, safe absorption.

Even related animals differ in their expression of the same disease. Most cats, domestic or exotic, develop kidney failure as they age. Some can live for years with this illness without showing signs, particularly the big cats from African and Asia. When a lion or tiger does become ill, it often responds well to a single treatment with fluids (under anesthesia, of course) and will feel better for months afterward. In contrast, cheetahs develop kidney failure at an earlier age and succumb to it more quickly, usually within a year.

In this final group of stories, zoo vets look to the experts in domestic animal and human medicine to diagnose and treat problems in various animals. Several seek help from talented medical professionals who willingly donate their expertise and time. The patients that benefit include a goldfish, a red kangaroo, a polar bear, a pair of weedy sea dragons, a giraffe calf, and a Nile hippo.

Lucy H. Spelman, DVM

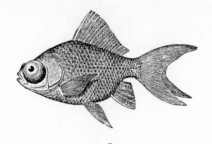

Tulip

by Greg Lewbart, MS, VMD

The corners of the stiff cardboard box were mashed and crinkled like so many miniature accordion bellows. When the UPS man slid the container across the cluttered counter, you could hear water sloshing back and forth, and the box rocked gently as its small internal waves pushed to break free.

"Initial on the X," the man said, handing me a clipboard. "Live fish, huh?"

"Well, I hope so," I said, scribbling my initials somewhere close to one of the many X's littering the sheet of paper. I handed the clipboard back. Instead of turning to leave, the UPS man looked anxiously at the box and then at me.

"When you gonna open it?"

"Right away," I said, surprised at his interest. "I'm going to open it right now."

I reached into my lab coat pocket for a pair of suture-removal scissors. They come in handy for all sorts of things, in addition to removing stitches. Holding them open and using one sharp edge, I sliced the wide piece of transparent tape along one edge of the box. I flipped back the large brown tabs to reveal several sheets of classified ads from the August 1993 *Des Moines Register*. At this point, the UPS man leaned over the box as if peering into a volcano. Tossing the newspaper aside, I snatched the double plastic bag from its cardboard hole. When I held the bag above my head so that the fluorescent ceiling light shone through it, we could both see an apple-sized orange-and-white blob swirling in the cool milky water. All that was left in the box was a perspiring, thawed ice pack.

"It's alive. Sure looks alive, anyway," the UPS man remarked.

"Yes. Yes, it is," I said with a smile. Then I addressed the fish, eye to unblinking eye. "Nice to meet you, Tulip."

"Tulip? You mean this fish has a name? Like it's some kinda pet?"

"Of course," I said to the startled deliveryman. I walked Tulip over to a running aquarium and floated her, bag and all, on the water's surface. This would help her acclimate to her new environment. Once she was safely afloat, I grabbed a blue plastic folder that had been lying next to the aquarium. "See. Here's her medical record."

"What's she got? What's she here for?"

"Probably has cancer," I said as I fiddled with the filter and checked the aquarium's water temperature. "Won't know for sure until we've run some tests."

"Cancer? Come on, Doc. Fish get cancer?"

"Absolutely. And older goldfish are especially prone to skin and muscle tumors." Then I pointed to what looked like a stem of cauliflower, dyed red, attached to the side of Tulip. "See this?"

By now the UPS man was standing with me, tank-side. "Yeah. That's cancer?"

"Well, like I said, we need to perform some diagnostic procedures. But it's most likely a tumor."

"Will she be all right?" he asked, with a degree of compassion that surprised me.

"Hard to tell. She's five years old and has survived two months of treatment with shark cartilage extract. Not to mention nearly twenty-four hours bouncing a thousand miles across the country in your box. Fish are pretty tough, though," I said. "We'll know a lot more tomorrow."

"Would it be all right if I check back in some day when I'm delivering? To see how the fish is?"

"Sure," I said. "She should be right here in this aquarium, unless she's in radiology or ultrasound having images made." Smiling, I added, "We have open visiting hours for fish patients."

Once Tulip was safely acclimated to her hospital tank, I picked up the phone to call Iowa. The woman who owned Tulip had tracked me down at North Carolina's veterinary school a few weeks ago, not an easy thing at the time. (This was before Google and the wide use of the Internet.) We'd talked several times about what to do next for this special fish, and I felt we'd made the right decision. Tulip seemed absolutely fine at the moment, despite her travels and her tumor. Dialing the number, I smiled at the thought of how her owner had found me.

A syndicated column called "News of the Weird" had run a short blurb about my work. Just above a paragraph headlined "Alien Abductees Form Support Group" was a short story about another fish, Zeus, I'd treated for a swim bladder disorder. The story, titled "Veterinarian Performs Surgery on Pet Fish," must have struck the editors as weird, though I certainly wasn't the only one working on pet fish in 1993. It spawned several morning rock-station interviews—there's a media service that feeds "odd" story fare to the radio networks—and apparently Tulip's owner heard one.

As I'd expected, she was relieved that Tulip had survived her overnight shipping ordeal and was anxious for my opinion of her pet's prognosis.

"It sure looks like a tumor," I said, trying to sound positive. "I'd like to take some radiographs and make sure it hasn't invaded the spine or any vital organs."

"You mean X-rays?" Tulip's owner said.

"Yes, exactly. And we might want to do an ultrasound too." I hesitated. "I would estimate that after these diagnostic tests, and a surgical biopsy of the tumor, your bill could run as high as four hundred dollars—"

"It doesn't matter what the cost is," she said, cutting me off. "Please do anything possible for her. Spare no expense."

"All right," I said. Her reaction didn't surprise me. An owner who commits to veterinary care for a pet fish by sending it UPS to an expert several states away is prepared to make a significant financial investment. I outlined the plan for the next twenty-four hours and we said our good-byes.

I looked over at Tulip. She was breathing comfortably with regularly expanding O-shaped lips. Then she moved her shiny white-and-orange globoid body to the rear of the tank and squirted out several hundred tiny fish eggs, a ritual she would practice on a daily basis while she was in my care. All mature female fish produce eggs. Some, like Tulip, will lay them even without the presence of a male (fertilization is external).

Tulip was as beautiful as the flower she was named for. At least until an ugly tumor started growing on her side. She was a five-year-old oranda goldfish—*Carassius auratus* to ichthyologists. Her ancestors all lived in Asia somewhere, and she was probably at least a twentieth-generation American. Her life began as a fertilized egg with about 150,000 siblings at a fish farm. Within a few months, she was moved to a tiny corner pet store in Iowa. Young fish, or fry, go through a lot during their first few months of life. Imagine a blur of nets, plastic bags, cardboard boxes, and loud motorized vehicles.

Tulip probably lived in a tank at the Iowa store with other fancy goldfish, the kind with strange-looking telescope eyes or big yellow sacs on the sides of their faces. No doubt, the store provided these fish with the basic amenities: plastic plants, colorful gravel, and one of those scuba divers that bobs up and down every few minutes. That guy would annoy me if I were a fish. If goldfish had teeth, they might try to bite through his air hose. Their teeth are in their throats, however. That's how they grind up hard pellets.

Fish do really like the gravel, though. It's like candy to

them. They suck up pieces of it, swirl it around in their mouths, and spit it out, swallowing the algae and bacterial slime that covers each little stone.

Tulip lived in the store for only about five weeks. Her owner spared no expense on a new aquarium, double the size of the group tank at the store. Gone were the plastic plants, diver, and dozens of other fish competing for food—and attention. Instead, Tulip swam among real plants. She had an automatic feeder that fed her the same time every day. Her weekly treats included a fresh pea or a freeze-dried worm.

According to her owner, Tulip had looked the picture of health until six months before, when the lump appeared on her side. It grew quickly, although if you looked at the fish from the healthy side, she appeared normal. From this description, I couldn't recommend the best course of treatment, so her owner agreed to send her all the way to North Carolina for a thorough exam.

Radiology was a breeze for Tulip and the hospital staff. She was the star patient of the day. No barking. No scratching. And no shedding! She lay on the plastic-covered X-ray plate like a big slimy dinner roll. Her breathing became more rapid out of water, but she didn't struggle at all. Once the technician had pushed the button to make the exposure, I was there to scoop her up and plop her back into her transport tank.

We took two views, one from the side and another from the top. The radiologist on duty marveled at their clarity and beauty. Fish radiographs always look beautiful to me. The delicate bones form a lacelike pattern. Aquatic animals have less bone density than a terrestrial animal of the same size. Tulip's two little otoliths (ear stones), used for balance in the water column, looked like small pearls in her head. Her pharyngeal teeth (the ones in the back of her throat) created rows of tiny white triangles.

Overall, Tulip's skeleton looked good, as did her egg-distended belly. And then there was the tumor. It had not spread into her spine or kidneys—very good news. This would also make surgery easier. Next stop, the operating room.

We anesthetized Tulip by placing her in a water bath containing a special fish anesthetic called MS-222. After about three minutes, she was asleep. The trick with this anesthesia is to keep the fish's gills submerged, adjusting the concentration of chemical in the water so the fish stays asleep. It sounds easy, but fish eyes are always wide open (no eyelids). You get used to it—your patient staring at you.

For Tulip's surgery, I was the anesthetist and my colleague, Dr. Craig Harms, performed the surgery. Craig is a reserved, humble, and extremely competent veterinarian with a soft, deep voice. Like a fuel-efficient automobile, he produces a lot from every word and action. He quietly accepted the challenge.

Our plan was to "debulk," or remove, as much of the tumor as we could. Craig used a technique called electrocautery, using a forcepslike device that cuts and controls bleeding at the same time. He quickly removed the tumor with very little bleeding. The entire procedure took less than fifteen minutes. To wake Tulip up, we flushed her gills with fresh water. In minutes, she was back in her tank, leaving us little egg presents.

We sent the tumor to the pathology laboratory and waited about forty-eight hours for the diagnosis. The results were grim: undifferentiated sarcoma. The fish had a malignancy that probably had not spread but was nonetheless an aggressive tumor. Even worse, we hadn't gotten it all. Repeating the surgery would do little at this stage. I informed Tulip's owner of the findings, and she agreed with me that our best recourse was to keep the fish in the hospital and consult with the university oncologist. If the UPS man wanted to stop by to see Tulip, he'd have plenty of time. (He never did. Maybe he didn't want to know the outcome.)

That's when Dr. David Ruslander entered the story. Dave is one of the most compassionate veterinarians I know. He's also one of the most opinionated. But the patient always came first. The arguments could wait for the bar or coffeehouse. Dave was thrilled to be involved with Tulip's case, and after carefully reviewing her medical record, radiographs, and biopsy report, he had a one-word suggestion: chemotherapy.

"I'm thinking cisplatin," Dave said with authority. "It's the best one for these nasty sarcomas. And I couldn't use radiation without frying the whole fish."

"But have you tried cisplatin on a fish?" I asked, virtually sure the answer was no. I also knew that this was a pretty heavy-duty drug with the potential for significant side effects in mammals.

"Nope," he said quickly. "And I don't imagine anyone else has, either. But if you don't go with the chemo, that thing's going to grow back. You don't have clean margins. And to get 'em you'd have to cut deep into the musculature."

"Yeah, I know," I said in a somber tone. "Well, I've got to talk with Tulip's owner. See what she says."

"No problem," he said, smiling. "We've got some time. But I wouldn't wait more than a couple of weeks."

Tulip stayed in the clinic aquarium for the next several weeks. She seemed fine, but close inspection of the surgery site revealed a small blip of tissue that was surely a new tumor. I showed this to Dave and he said simply, "It's cisplatin or more surgery. Or both."

"Both?"

"Well, with this aggressive a tumor, the chemo might not be enough," Dave said.

Unfortunately, Dave's prediction was accurate. Tulip was tranquilized for an injection of the cisplatin. We used an anesthetic just to take the edge off, which she tolerated well. But the tumor continued to grow during the next several weeks. Craig performed a second, more aggressive surgery, which cut into the underlying muscle. Tulip tolerated the second surgery well, which was followed a week later by a second and final round of injectable chemotherapy. But still the tumor persisted.

"I think my baby's had enough, don't you?" Tulip's mom said to me through hundreds of miles of phone line. "I mean, will more surgery or chemo stop this thing?"

"I don't know. We're sort of in uncharted territory," I said.

"Maybe we should just let it run its course," she said. "She looks a lot better than she did, right?"

"Right," I said, perking up a bit. "She certainly looks better. And she's still eating well and laying eggs."

"Well, maybe it's time to send her home. Can you do that?"

"Yes, of course. We'll pack her up and send her home this week."

I don't think I ever had a more nervous night. Visions of Tulip's box falling off a truck or being misplaced in some dark warehouse cluttered my mind from the time I closed the lid to the time I got the phone call the next afternoon. Tulip had made it home safely! Once again, she caught the attention of the UPS man—the one in Iowa. Tulip's owner sent me a photo of the deliveryman holding the box with the fish, flowers, balloons, and a "Welcome Home, Tulip!" sign.

Maybe we could have tried something more or something different to help this beautiful fish. Her case motivated us to find a new approach: we now use laser surgery to remove these tumors. But at the time, we felt as if we'd exhausted all possibilities. The tumor would undoubtedly shorten Tulip's life, but the fish would be back with her loving owner. I imagined the goldfish relaxed and happy, swimming again in her roomy tank and eating bits of fresh peas.

ABOUT THE AUTHOR

Gregory A. Lewbart graduated from Gettysburg College in 1981 with a bachelor's degree in biology; he received his master's degree in biology from Northeastern University in 1985. In 1988 he graduated from the University of Pennsylvania School of Veterinary Medicine. Dr. Lewbart worked for a large wholesaler of ornamental fishes before joining the faculty at the North Carolina State University College of Veterinary Medicine in 1993, where he is a professor of aquatic animal medicine. Board certified by the American College of Zoological Medicine, he is the author of over ninety popular and scientific articles about invertebrates, fish, amphibians, and reptiles, as well as the first textbook on invertebrate medicine. Dr. Lewbart has also written two novels, *Ivory Hunters* (1996) and *Pavilion Key* (2000), both scientific mysteries that address issues of wildlife conservation and man's exploitation of the environment. He and his wife, Dr. Diane Deresienski, also a veterinarian, live in Raleigh with their assorted pets.

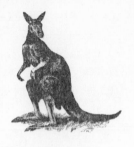

Empathy

by Roberto Aguilar, DVM

When we first examined Sally the kangaroo, she lay in shock on the ground. Her pupils were dilated and she showed no response to people approaching or touching her. She seemed unable to use her rear legs and lacked muscle tone around her cloaca (the combined rectal-and-bladder opening found in all marsupials). She could move her front legs in what appeared to be a coordinated manner, however.

The two rambunctious emus that had chased the mob of kangaroos, sending Sally crashing into the fence, stood quietly at the far end of the exhibit. These birds often chased the kangaroos—and each other. During particularly active chases, the kangaroos could really get going. This wasn't the first time the emus had done damage.

In their native Australia, red kangaroos live in wide open

grasslands where their strong, heavy lower bodies are an advantage. Deerlike eyes and ears give this odd and interesting species a delicate look. In fact, they are very hardy in most circumstances. Their powerful rear legs and tails give them the option of fight or flight. They can stand up to box, kick out at predators, or hop at breakneck speed. If excited, they will explode into action.

In the wild, however, they don't often encounter the tough and impenetrable obstacle of a chain-link fence. Excited zoo kangaroos may simply circle in their pen, or they may make a break for it through the fence. It's an unfortunate but common choice, given that the animal is hell-bent on fleeing. Usually the outcome is nothing worse than a very surprised and dazed kangaroo. If they hit the fence face-on, though, the impact on their upper body is huge. Sometimes they suffer severe neck injuries.

Over the years, we'd had two such cases at the Audubon Zoo in New Orleans, where I worked as staff veterinarian. We found the animals down and unable to move. Spinal injuries are not situations that can be treated easily even in domestic animals, let alone kangaroos. Our success rate so far was zero.

We moved Sally carefully to the zoo's hospital. A systematic neurological exam showed us that the injury was most likely in the spinal cord, our worst fear.

We took radiographs of her neck and chest and found that her second and third vertebrae were out of place. Because the spinal cord is not visible on a plain X-ray, we did a myelogram next. This test involves injecting a special dye into the space around the spinal cord and taking a series of radiographs so that we can see the precise site of damage. Normally the dye moves quickly down the length of the cord and fills the space evenly. In this case, the dye marking the outline of the spinal cord narrowed just at the point where the bones looked out of alignment.

In a way, this result was a good sign. The damage had occurred at a single point along the spinal cord, involving just two adjacent neck vertebrae and not the fragile first one. All marsupials have a uniquely shaped first cervical vertebra—the first bone in the neck under the skull. These bones have deep central indentations in kangaroos, making them wing-shaped and therefore somewhat unstable. At least Sally's first vertebra had not been damaged.

We knew right away whom to call: our consulting neurosurgeon, Dr. Mitchell Harris. He might be able to realign those two bones surgically and allow the pinched nerve tissue to heal. If anyone could give Sally a chance to recover, he could. I dialed him immediately.

Like most zoos, we kept a long list of specialists—a mixture of veterinarians and physicians—willing to help us out with difficult cases. The choice of whether to call a human or an animal doctor depended largely on the problem. In this case, we called a physician because of his exceptional skill. Dr. Harris was simply the best in the region at dealing with spinal injuries in any species, human or otherwise.

Luckily for us, he was in town and available. With his usual enthusiasm, he offered to help us organize what we'd need to work on the injured kangaroo. Though he directed an orthopedic trauma and spinal surgery center for humans, it didn't seem to matter that this new patient had four legs and a thick tail. Within hours, we had assembled an entire team of specialists and equipment and scheduled the surgery for the next morning, which would allow the kangaroo time to stabilize and the experts to gather.

Early the next morning, Sally's condition appeared about the same—neither worse nor better. She'd spent a quiet night in our intensive care unit in a small, warmed cage. To reduce the swelling in her spinal cord, we gave her intravenous fluids along with some steroids. Unlike a healthy kangaroo that would kick and bounce around in a confined space, she needed no sedation because she couldn't move.

Dr. Harris arrived at the clinic early. He brought with him a full set of specialized tools, a surgical nurse, and another physician to assist during surgery. We were also joined by another veterinarian, an anesthesiologist from the nearest veterinary school two hours north, Louisiana State University School of Veterinary Medicine. Together we reviewed the X-rays and myelogram. Dr. Harris decided on a surgical approach through the back of Sally's neck.

About an hour later, the kangaroo lay on her stomach under anesthesia, ready for the surgery to begin. We placed her head on a rolled towel, allowing her neck to rest in a natural position. We clipped away a large patch of fur and scrubbed the area for surgery. With a scalpel, Dr. Harris made a vertical incision in the skin, starting just above the base of the neck. Next he used scissors and forceps to bluntly dissect between the muscles, tracing the path of each one to identify its function. Using tiny clawlike clamps, he pulled the muscle fibers off to one side as he slowly worked deeper. His goal was to get down to the affected bones without damaging the muscles. This was a painstaking process, and the fact that nobody had ever done it before in a kangaroo made it slow going.

In terms of surgical anatomy, we had few bipedal mammals to use for comparison. Dr. Harris frequently asked us what was normal and what was not. He pointed to a place where one of the neck muscles split in two. Was that normal anatomy, or had it occurred when the kangaroo hit the fence? We really didn't know. No textbooks existed for the kangaroo spine.

Fortunately, many aspects of anatomy and surgery are universal among mammals. For example, both kangaroos and humans have cartilage lining the articular surfaces (facets) between the vertebral wings and cartilaginous discs between the vertebral bodies. Both have ligaments holding the vertebrae in alignment, tendons that attach bone to muscle, and muscles crossing the surfaces of multiple vertebrae to give the spinal column strength. And in any species, the rate of post-operative healing depends on the degree of tissue damage and the quality of the blood supply to the affected area.

With these principles in mind, Dr. Harris was diligent, careful, and delicate, extrapolating from his experience in humans to preserve the normal anatomy and blood supply while making his way down to the misaligned bones. After half an hour, the affected vertebrae had been exposed with minimal bleeding. That in itself was an amazing feat.

Then came the most difficult, risky part of the procedure: realigning the spinal canal. In pushing the vertebrae back into their original positions, we faced one of two outcomes. We could successfully align the spinal canal and remove the pressure on the cord, allowing the damaged nerves a chance to heal. Or we could align the bones but in the process damage the cord further by increasing the trauma and bleeding in the area.

Carefully, and still ever so slowly, Dr. Harris pushed the vertebrae back into their original positions with his skillful hands. We heard a slight pop. Everyone held his or her breath except for the anesthetized Sally, who continued to breathe normally. A good sign, given that any manipulation of the spinal cord can disrupt descending signals from the brain. Nothing seemed to have worsened, so we continued the procedure.

After placing the spinal canal in what we hoped would be its normal position, Dr. Harris drilled small steel pins through the spinal processes of the second and third vertebrae. He wired the pins to each other and across the top, forming an H-shaped pattern. "It's known as a modified Dewar's technique," he explained. The repair held both vertebrae firmly in place.

Next, we used bone cement to reinforce the pins and wire, knowing we couldn't ask the kangaroo to sit still and stay in bed for a couple of months. We considered a bone graft to add support, but rejected the idea for the same reason. She needed complete, or near-complete, stability the moment she woke up. Her first hop, no matter how soft, would send vibrations right up to the unstable area. A bone graft would take weeks to solidify. We questioned whether the bone cement, the kind used to secure a new hip joint in a human, would be strong enough in the long run, but it was our only option.

During the entire procedure, Dr. Harris had remained calm, methodical, and relaxed. Even during tense moments, his voice and manner remained steady. When he removed his mask after the surgery, he looked pleased as he surveyed his handiwork. I guessed that he saw the entire effort as fairly routine. He simply applied what he already knew to a different species. To me, it was nothing short of a small miracle.

Dr. Harris knelt down next to the kangaroo while she woke up from the anesthesia. Watching the two of them, I noticed a linear scar crossing the back of the neurosurgeon's neck. My mind came to an instant conclusion, confirmed months later when I finally got up the nerve to ask: the doctor had undergone a similar surgical procedure years earlier. Maybe that's why he'd become an expert in this field.

Sally lay on her side, shivering as the anesthetic wore off. It would be some time before we knew if the kangaroo could use her limbs. We'd taken radiographs at the end of the procedure and everything looked good—in perfect alignment. Nevertheless, we could not be certain she still had nerve function.

I saw the surgeon's clinical expression soften into a look of gentle, benevolent concern. It lasted only briefly—a few seconds—and then he smiled. From then on, I knew that Sally would be a patient our kind surgeon would never forget. He had felt what she felt.

Animals often represent more to us than their simple selves. Every patient deserves our empathy and compassion. Many also earn our respect, affection, or sympathy for a variety of reasons. We often try to control these emotions when they surface, as Dr. Harris did while working on Sally. Too much feeling can get in the way of good medicine. Too much worry about what the animal is feeling can draw your attention away from the task at hand. Alternatively, too little makes it impossible to do your best.

Sally made a relatively rapid and complete recovery. It was not easy, but we kept her in a heavily bedded and padded recovery stall, much like the ones used for horses recovering from anesthesia. Four heavy pads covered the walls, preventing the animal from hurting herself if she stumbled trying to sit up or stand. The abundant straw bedding helped make the kangaroo comfortable. By the third day she had recovered movement in her legs and tone in her cloaca. Her appetite picked up and she accepted all of her food treats.

Over the following weeks, Sally became stronger and her movements gained coordination. We often looked in on her, only to find her looking curiously back at us while munching on a piece of hay. For her physical therapy, we helped her to her feet and held her tail while she hopped in place. After thirty days in our hospital, she could stand for several minutes at a time. After ninety days, she had completely recovered. We walked the kangaroo into a large plastic kennel and took her back to the exhibit.

For years afterward, I offered Dr. Harris an update every time I saw him. I'd describe how well the kangaroo was doing on exhibit. She appeared healthy and active, indistinguishable from the others. Dr. Harris would smile broadly and say, "Of course she's fantastic. She's Sally!"

Our neurosurgeon, a physician and scientist, took a great leap in this case. He allowed himself to identify with a kangaroo. I'd like to see that kind of emotional crossover into the animal kingdom happen more often.

ABOUT THE AUTHOR

Born and raised in Mexico City, Mexico, Roberto F. Aguilar graduated from the National Autonomous University of Mexico in 1987. He did an internship in veterinary medicine at Oklahoma State University and a clinical residency in orthopedic avian surgery at the University of Minnesota. He served as staff veterinarian and then senior veterinarian at the Audubon Zoo in New Orleans from 1992 to 2005 and is currently director of conservation and science at the Phoenix Zoo. The author of numerous publications, including a book on exotic animal medicine, Dr. Aguilar has lectured extensively in most of Latin America and is the manager for Latinvets, a Listserv with more than 600 members in Latin America, Europe, and the United States.

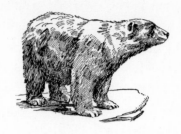

Polar Bears STAT

by Jennifer Langan, DVM

I was preparing for the day's cases when I heard over the radio, "Any 500 veterinary unit, 10-76 polar bear dens *stat*!" At Chicago's Brookfield Zoo, our vet hospital call number is 500. The urgent message directed that any and all zoo vets go straight (called 10-76) to the polar bear grottoes. Since I was the only one working that day, that meant me.

Running out the door, I called to our two vet students to follow. This would be a learning experience for them, no matter what the problem was. We sped across the park to assess the situation. The polar bear keepers met me at the entrance to the dens and took me to see Aussie, down a long, cavelike, cement-floored corridor to the inside holding dens. Despite the rising summer heat outside, the cool, moist air carried the unmistakable smell of bear—a strong musty odor. Aussie, our twenty-year-old male breeding polar bear, stood at the cage front. He had a very large swelling, about half the size of a basketball, protruding from his belly button.

I bent down to look at him through thick iron bars, so that the big polar bear and I were face-to-face. He was obviously in extreme discomfort, legs splayed, swaying back and forth with the biggest hernia I had ever seen. Aussie needed emergency surgery.

I'd repaired hernias before, but never in such a large patient. The students searched the literature about hernia repair in bears, finding very little. I spoke to a vet at another zoo who'd done a similar—and successful—surgery on their polar bear. It helped to know that we wouldn't be the first to attempt this procedure and that we could use a standard domestic-animal surgical approach. Moving Aussie to and from the operating room presented the biggest challenge.

I decided to call the vet school for help. Unlike zoo vets, veterinary surgeons operate daily and repair hernias often. They don't work on bears, of course, but this was not a bear-specific problem. Any species can develop a hernia. I'd anesthetize Aussie by dart, we'd move him to the hospital clinic for the surgery, and the experts would take it from there. They'd extrapolate using techniques established for domestic animals. The operation would go faster, and I'd be able to focus my attention on the logistics of working on a polar bear.

Four hours later, we were ready to start. A veterinary surgeon and an anesthesiologist from the University of Illinois at Urbana-Champaign College of Veterinary Medicine were on their way. Our vet techs had prepped the large-animal surgery room for a thousand-pound patient. The chief of police had organized an escort; the zoo's forklift driver was on his way. A crowd of keepers, assistant curators, and curators had gathered to help.

Earlier, I'd contemplated the best choice of anesthetic agents for this older, compromised polar bear. Patient safety, the safety of all the staff who would be helping to carry the bear, and the safety of the visitors in the park were all of equal concern. Polar bears are extremely dangerous animals, smart and quick, one of nature's most powerful carnivores. If I miscalculated the amount of drug needed and Aussie woke up from his anesthesia during transport across the zoo grounds on a busy summer day, we would have a serious problem. There isn't an anesthetic dart that would work fast enough. In that case, our zoo police force had the authority to shoot to kill our patient.

This is a part of our emergency response plan I hope never to see implemented during my career. But like all zoos, we have policies in place to ensure human as well as animal safety. I briefed the group on the potential dangers involved. We needed to take every precaution and work together as a team.

Pushing the possibility of disaster out of my mind, I picked up my darting kit and walked down the hall to the den. As I approached the cage, Aussie finally sat down and let me have a good look at his belly. About five years earlier, the polar bear had developed a golf-ball–sized fatty swelling at his navel, a small umbilical hernia that was hard to see even in strong light. It hadn't changed in years, nor had it caused Aussie any discomfort—until today. Now the hernia was impossible to miss. The area was hugely swollen.

When we first noticed the hernia, we'd anesthetized Aussie for ultrasound examination and physical palpation to confirm our diagnosis. The cause of this problem is usually a small amount of fatty tissue caught in the area around the umbilical cord (belly button) at birth, creating a small opening in the muscles in the middle of the abdominal wall. If this hole enlarges over time, organs like the intestines can follow.

Many small umbilical hernias never change during the life of the patient, so they are monitored rather than removed surgically unless the animal shows signs of pain or the swelling changes in size. If this happens, the chances are that more than fat is wedged in the area. It can be a life-threatening condition, particularly when it happens acutely.

Usually, by this time in the morning, Aussie would be banging on the door to be given access to his outside exhibit and pool. Today he had no such interest. He was vocalizing and panting at the front of his cage. I darted Aussie with a combination of anesthetic agents (medetomidine and tiletamine-zolazepam) in his right front shoulder. He hardly reacted, probably distracted by the discomfort from his hernia. Within about fifteen minutes, the polar bear lay on his side, eyes partially closed, breathing deeply.

It was my responsibility to make sure that Aussie was really asleep and that he would stay that way until we could hook him up to gas anesthesia for surgery. One of the assets of bear dens is their solid, bunkerlike construction, which helps them maintain comfortable constant temperatures for the animals. But that construction also means the doorways are small, requiring humans to bend down and negotiate a large cement step to get in and out. I crawled into the den slowly, hoping to find a deeply anesthetized polar bear while also contemplating my what-if plan.

Fortunately, the anesthetic drugs had done their job. With the help of about twenty keepers, I was able to roll Aussie onto a cargo net, lift him through the narrow doorway (no easy feat), and heave him onto a wooden pallet. Aussie was so large that his head and legs still hung over all sides of the polar-bear–sized stretcher we had constructed earlier that day. The forklift slowly picked him up and backed down the long, dimly lit access hall to where a flatbed truck awaited us. Though security staff had roped off our immediate work area, a large crowd of spectators had gathered, recognizing that something out of the ordinary was transpiring.

For the ride through the zoo grounds, I climbed up onto the flatbed to monitor the bear's anesthesia. The flatbed was a narrow space with low wooden sidewalls, barely wide enough for both of us. Wedged between the wet, smelly bear and the wall, I felt a rush of adrenaline when Aussie voluntarily moved one of his huge paws. It had only been a short time since I'd darted him. Maybe he wasn't as deeply asleep as I'd thought? I gave him an additional amount of anesthetic intravenously using a vein in his rear leg. Thankfully, it worked quickly. A few minutes later, we were ready to begin our trip from the bear dens to the vet hospital.

Our zoo is a beautifully planted park with winding pathways leading from one animal exhibit to another——but no back access road. We had no choice but to drive right through the park, slowly. Zoo police cleared the way as we drove. A crowd of several hundred people watched as we wound our way from the bear exhibit to Roosevelt Fountain, past the back side of Tropic World, and finally off the grounds and out of sight. Our supersized patient slept through it all.

At the hospital, we inserted a breathing tube normally used for fifteen-hundred-pound horses into Aussie's airway so that we could administer gas anesthesia during the surgery. We placed intravenous catheters attached to fluid lines in order to administer preoperative antibiotics, fluids, and pain medication. The polar bear's entire belly was shaved and scrubbed with antiseptic solution, revealing the black skin under his white fur—normal for polar bears. We rolled him into surgery and positioned him on his back with all four legs and neck extended. Earlier, I'd asked carpenters to reinforce the surgery table so it could handle Aussie's unusual weight and size, and to my relief the emergency modifications held.

Soon a great many blue surgical drapes covered all of Aussie's body except the area of the distended hernia. The specialists from the veterinary school went right to work. Dr. Rachael Carpenter helped monitor anesthesia while Dr. Chris Byron got started on the surgery. He began with an incision in front of the hernia in order to feel inside Aussie's abdomen to see if there were intestines or a piece of the spleen or other organ trapped within the swelling. If this was the case, a longer and more difficult surgery would be required, and Aussie's health would be at greater risk.

The danger is that when these tissues squeeze through the small hernia opening, their blood supply can be compromised; this can result in death of the tissue and severe infection in a patient, particularly when loops of intestine are involved. Sometimes the damaged intestine must also be removed, a surgery known as a bowel resection. Fortunately, this was not the case. The herniated tissue consisted only of fat. The object of the surgery was relatively simple: expose the hole in the muscle, remove the herniated fat, and suture the rent in the abdominal wall so it never splits open again.

To access the area, Dr. Byron incised the skin in an elliptical fashion on both sides of the hernia using electrocautery to control any bleeding. Over the next hour, he removed several pounds of traumatized skin and subcutaneous tissue from the hernia site, as well as a large amount of necrotic (dead) fat. The actual defect through which the abdominal fat had squeezed to form the swelling was surprisingly small, only about four inches long. Once the edges of the hernia had been sutured to close the hole, the site was lavaged with saline. Then the surgeon closed the subcutaneous fat and tissue in three separate layers, a technique designed to hold the weight of Aussie's heavy belly when he stood up. Finally, the skin was closed with absorbable stitches to spare us from having to remove them at a later date.

We moved our patient back to his den at around seven PM in the same way he'd been brought to the hospital. Though the logistics were easier this time and the commute much quicker, the drive back was still a bit scary: by now it was dark, requiring us to monitor the bear's anesthesia with flashlights. Back in the den, I stayed with Aussie until he woke up, acutely aware that I was once again jammed in a small space—about the size of my bathroom—with one of North America's largest and most dangerous carnivores. Fortunately, Aussie woke up slowly and quietly, a smooth recovery that gave me plenty of time to exit safely. Tired and filthy, I got to my feet, heaved a sigh of relief, and thanked everyone for their extraordinary efforts. All the planning and preparation had paid off.

I hoped Aussie would feel a whole lot better soon. But the next morning, the polar bear refused to eat, drink, and take his medicine. We'd prescribed oral pain medication and antibiotics. He paced and panted. The keepers tempted him with all his favorite foods (bread, fish, and meat) to no avail. Even normally forbidden treats like soft-serve ice cream, jelly donuts, and honey failed. He wanted absolutely nothing to do with any of us.

I hated to antagonize him after what he'd been through the day before, but I had no choice except to dart him with his medication. If infection was brewing, we needed to control it with antibiotics. And if we could control the pain he must be feeling after the two-and-a-half-hour surgery, he might feel like eating and drinking. This time Aussie reacted to being darted with a roar so loud I seemed to feel it as well as hear it. It was a sound that echoed through the cavernous access tunnels and could probably be heard throughout the park. Thank goodness I didn't have to crawl through a small doorway into his den today.

By the following morning, Aussie had improved. Although I was happy to see him feeling better, he was not at all happy to see me. He looked me up and down and from side to side, as if to see if I'd brought along another dart for him. Sadly, our patients often hold a grudge against us. We try so hard to help them, and then they remember us with fear, even hatred—strong emotions to assign to a bear, but certainly the impression Aussie gave at that moment. Nonetheless, he was soon eating and interacting with his keepers. They were still his friends.

Though the surgery had been accomplished successfully, I still had a major concern: would the suture at Aussie's hernia site hold up to the weight of his immense belly? After all, suture material is not designed with half-ton polar bears in mind. In the case of a large domestic animal, a belly bandage could be placed around the abdomen to support it and keep the wound clean. There was no way this would be possible with a polar bear. We'd just have to do our best to see that the surgery site stayed clean and that he didn't overexert himself.

Healthy polar bears are very active and spend much of their day walking or swimming. After recuperating in his den for over two weeks, Aussie began to go stir-crazy. He started banging on the door to let the keepers know he wanted access outside. Since his incision appeared healed, with no evidence of infection or hernia recurrence, we gave him a clean bill of health; it was time for him to go back on exhibit. The moment the door was opened, Aussie rushed out and headed straight for, you guessed it, the pool—just where you'd imagine a polar bear would go on a hot summer day. He hit the ice-cold water with a bounding belly flop, of course.

ABOUT THE AUTHOR

Jennifer Langan has had a lifelong interest in both free-ranging and captive wildlife. After earning a bachelor's degree in animal science at the Agricultural College of the University of Illinois, she completed her studies at its

College of Veterinary Medicine. Dr. Langan did a small animal internship at Angell Memorial Animal Hospital in Boston and a residency in zoological medicine at the University of Tennessee, and then completed a fellowship with the Conservation Medicine Center of Chicago at Brookfield Zoo. Board certified by the American College of Zoological Medicine in 2001, she subsequently joined the faculty at the University of Illinois, where she is now an assistant clinical professor. Dr. Langan cofounded the Chicago Zoological and Aquatic Animal Residency Program, of which she is one of the directors. She spends the majority of her time as a clinical veterinarian working with students and residents at Brookfield Zoo.

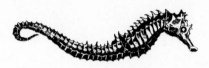

Water-Breathing Dragons
by Ilze Berzins, PhD, DVM

Alex walked into my office with a frown on his face. "Dr. Berzins, we're in trouble. The dragons are floating."

"What do you mean?!" I asked, trying not to panic. These are not words you want to hear about any new fish shipment, especially when the transport box contains a pair of rare weedy sea dragons, the first to arrive at your aquarium.

"They're at the surface and can't seem to dive down."

A sea dragon is not, as the name suggests, the size of the Loch Ness Monster. It is a delicate, unusual-looking, and endangered fish from Australia, related to the sea horse, the tiny S-shaped fish you can buy almost anywhere. Dragons have elaborate leafy appendages, like fronds of seaweed, attached to their colorful bodies. At most, a full-grown weedy sea dragon reaches eighteen inches in length and weighs less than three ounces.

Everyone on staff at the Florida Aquarium had been excited about the arrival of these special fish. In one way or another, we'd all helped in the planning, which had taken over a year, starting in the spring of 1998. As the aquarium's head of veterinary services, I'd been involved in every step of the preparations. Our biologists had researched ideal water conditions, housing, and what to feed the fish. Using this information, our exhibit designers had custom-built a new tank, one that would also provide a great view of the dragons for aquarium guests. Our marketing and public relations people had taken it from there, naming the new exhibit Dragons Down Under. I'd talked to a number of other fish vets about dragon medicine, just in case something went wrong.

The dragons had arrived at the aquarium that morning via special air cargo from Melbourne, Australia, with a stopover in Los Angeles. We'd planned that the fish would stay in a special holding tank for a minimum thirty-day quarantine. This would give them time to recover from the stress of transport. We'd also check them for parasites, deworm them if necessary, and keep a close eye on their feeding behavior. Next we'd move them to the new exhibit if they were healthy.

Given their long plane flight and the two days they'd spent in a dark, sealed bag, I fully expected to find one or both of the dragons acting sluggish or looking thin. These are common signs of mild stress due to shipping, since fish are not fed during transport and are in a confined space.

At worst, if the concentration of dissolved oxygen in the

water had dropped more than it should have, or if a consider-able level of nitrogen (the waste product of fish) had accu-mulated, I wouldn't have been surprised if the dragons had a high gilling rate. This sign of stress is equivalent to breathing fast. By rapidly opening and closing their gills, which are sup-plied by a dense network of capillaries, fish can take in more oxygen and also get rid of waste products that build up in the bloodstream.

Alex, one of our biologists, held the lid of the box open while I took my first look at the dragons. Just as he'd warned, they were floating at the surface and struggling to stay up-right. I watched them for several minutes, thinking about what to do next. For whatever reason, they couldn't keep their bodies beneath the water's surface. This species of sea dragon has a long snout, and the gills sit right behind the angle of the jaw. Neither of the new dragons could keep its snout or gills under the water. They were piping, or gasping—not for air, but for water. This was a life-threatening situation. No vertebrate animal can survive with-out oxygen. Something must have gone wrong during the shipment, or perhaps the box hadn't been properly prepared to begin with.

I quickly directed Alex to take a sample of the shipment water to the water quality lab. He'd been instrumental in helping me get the animals to Florida, following up on every detail to make certain everything went smoothly. He looked just as worried about the dragons as I was. We tested for tem-perature, nitrogen waste product levels such as ammonia and nitrite, dissolved oxygen saturation, salinity, and pH. The re-sults were normal.

If the problem wasn't in the water, it had to be inside the patients. Dragons, like many other types of fish, have air bladders (also called gas or swim bladders). This organ helps them with buoyancy control, so that they can maintain their position in the water. Maybe their air bladders had become overinflated during transport. Even worse, they might have ruptured, allowing free air into their body cavities. This excess air, whether inside the bladder or outside, would make it impossible for the fish to swim beneath the surface of the water.

I ran through the possible reasons for an overinflated air bladder. Changes in air pressure during the flight could cause this; maybe the cargo hold hadn't been properly pressurized. The lower pressure could result in gas leaving the bloodstream and forming gas bubbles in the tissues of the fish. Another possibility was that the box had been exposed to excessively low temperatures, which could have affected the concentration of oxygen and other gases in the water and bloodstream, increasing the amount of gas released into the air bladder, and then expanding when temperatures warmed up again. Or, and this last possibility was at the top of my rule-out list, the water in the sealed transport bag had been supersaturated with oxygen gas during some part of their trip.

If you've ever purchased a pet fish for your home aquarium, you may have seen the salesperson tie the plastic bag so that it puffs out with air, like a half-filled water balloon. The oxygen in the air will help keep the oxygen levels in the water at a healthy level. When fish are transported long distances, pressurized oxygen gas is added to the container to ensure that oxygen levels remain high inside the bag for several days. But if the dragons' sealed bag was inadvertently overpressurized, the gas pressure inside the air space, and thus the water, would have been initially too high, exposing the dragons to excessive, harmful gas pressures.

It was going to be difficult, if not impossible, to find out for certain what had happened to the dragons during transport, and it wouldn't necessarily change the treatment options. Time was of the essence. My priority was to confirm the diagnosis even if I couldn't be certain of the root cause. The game plan was simple: radiograph the animals to look for overinflated air bladders.

Since the dragons were small and relatively inactive, they didn't need anesthesia for radiography. We could position them on the X-ray film cassettes the way we do other small fish, take the picture quickly, and replace them in the water. Gently I picked up the first patient, wearing powderless latex gloves to minimize damage to its skin and protective mucus, and placed it on its side directly onto the cassette. Susan, my veterinary technician, positioned the X-ray beam, lined everything up, and set the machine. She got ready to hit the exposure button while I darted behind the lead screen. Seconds later, I ran back into the room to return the dragon to the water. We repeated the procedure for our second patient.

After developing the film, we could see that the body cavity of one dragon was completely filled with air. In the other, we saw the outline of an overinflated air bladder, which was most likely compressing the intestines directly below the bladder.

There might appear to be a simple solution to this life-

threatening problem: place a needle into the air bladder and
withdraw the excess air. But in a sea dragon, such a procedure can result in the introduction of infections or in laceration of other internal organs. To complicate matters further,
the dragons' thick scales, like a coat of bony armor, make it
difficult to insert a needle through the skin without squashing
the fish.

I had another idea: treat the fish as you would a human. Put
them in a high-pressure chamber that gradually moves the
trapped gas out of the wrong places. Maybe we could take
them to a dive chamber and treat them as if they had the
bends, a common complication of scuba diving. Florida is a
popular diving destination, and I knew there were several recompression chambers nearby.

This thinking was based on what we know about fish
anatomy. The air bladder is normally filled with various
gases, oxygen being one of them, thanks to a system known
as countercurrent exchange. The oxygen gets there via a
complex bed of arterial and venous capillaries known as the
rete mirabile (Latin for "wonderful net"). The capillaries are
arranged in such a manner that blood rich in oxygen flows
past blood low in oxygen; the gas then moves from areas of
high to low concentration. The exchange takes place near the
wall of the air bladder, so it can deflate or inflate depending
on the concentration of the gases passing by in the blood vessels. By exposing the dragons to high pressure, simulating a
dive, maybe we could drive the gas back out of the bladder
and into the bloodstream.

Fish also use countercurrent exchange to breathe. The
arrangement of capillaries in the gills is not as elaborate as in

the swim bladder rete, but the overall result is the same. The gas moves from high to low concentration, from the water into the bloodstream and then to the tissues. This is, of course, why our floating dragons were in big trouble. Their overinflated air bladders prevented them from keeping their gills underwater. If we could get the gas out of the air bladder and into the bloodstream, maybe it could leave via the gills.

Though we humans don't have an air bladder, the gases in our bloodstream are subject to the same rules of physics. They move in and out according to pressure as well as chemical differences. The bends, also known as decompression sickness, occurs when scuba divers ascend too quickly. The air in their tanks has been compressed under pressure, ensuring that oxygen is delivered to the tissue as they dive down. As long as the diver ascends slowly, these gases will leave the body as the pressure equalizes. However, if the diver rises to the surface too fast, the gases will expand and form bubbles in blood vessels and tissues, which can cause painful tissue damage or even death. Trapped gas in the wrong place is a medical emergency—in any species.

I decided to go for it. It sounded like a weird plan, taking tiny fish that look like seaweed into a hospital recompression chamber, but why not give it a try? I knew that our local hospital, St. Joseph's, had such a chamber. In addition to treating dive accidents, it's used in the treatment of several human diseases, including diabetes. People with this disease have very poor circulation in their feet and hands, and the increased chamber pressure helps improve oxygenation.

For people with the bends, the chamber pressure forces

gas bubbles in the tissues to dissolve and go back into the bloodstream, where the gas would then be slowly released out through the lungs. In the case of the sea dragons, I hoped for the same thing: the pressure would compress the excess gas out of the air bladder and allow it to be absorbed back into the bloodstream, and out of the body through the gills.

When I called the hospital, the officials responded to my odd request by giving us an appointment for the next morning. Because running the chamber is time-consuming and expensive, they requested that the dragons share the chamber with several human patients. Grateful for the offer, and knowing the dragons couldn't survive for much longer, I accepted.

In order to keep the animals from staying at the surface overnight, we placed them in the container we'd prepared for their arrival. Using a plastic grate, we gently pushed the dragons down into the water and left the grate in place so that they would remain several inches under the surface.

The next morning, Alex filled a portable acrylic tank with about twenty gallons of water and set it in a shallow Styrofoam container to which we added ice. We wanted the water temperature in the tank to stay relatively cool, around 60° Fahrenheit. He added an air stone attached to a small portable compressed air tank that would keep the water oxygenated. Carefully I slipped the animals into the tank and, with the help of Alex and three other biologists, slowly lifted the "travel package" into a van.

An entourage of officials and public relations personnel met us at the hospital. Dragon paparazzi!! The local press wanted to film the event because it was so unusual; also because it helped highlight the fact that many of the procedures used in human medicine can be applicable to animals (in fact, many are first developed using animals).

We set the tank and accessories on a cart and wheeled it down the hall to the chamber room. The chamber itself looked like a large steel bank vault, with pressurized windows on the sides, and several chairs. There were lots of curious looks as well as a few chuckles from the hospital staff and the human patients who were waiting for the procedure to start. Maybe the sea creatures would help make a long, boring procedure a bit more exciting for everyone. After the people had taken their places in the chamber, I walked in with the tank that held the dragons and set it near one of the windows so Alex and I could watch the procedure.

The hatch was closed, locked, and sealed to deal with the pressure changes, and the process began. The pressure in the chamber would slowly increase, simulating a sixty-foot dive. The two animals in the acrylic tank gradually began to sink toward the bottom—precisely as we had hoped. There were a few thumbs-up gestures from the patients in the chamber. *Phew,* I thought, *maybe we can save these little guys after all.*

For the next few hours, there was nothing for us to do but wait and hope the capillary beds inside the sea dragons could do their jobs. As we waited, we talked with hospital staff and the patients' relatives about aquatic animal medicine. They were amazed at what was possible. We explained that we routinely take fish radiographs, perform surgery, and treat a range of different animals, from corals to sharks. We even use many of the same antibiotics and other drugs used in

people. The range of success, however, is variable: aquatic
medicine is still a new frontier in veterinary medicine.

When time was up, we watched anxiously as the pressure
in the chamber was slowly reduced. At about thirty feet, the
sea dragons gradually moved upward, but not all the way.
Holding my own breath, I hoped they would hold their positions. But as soon as the pressure returned to room conditions, the animals were back on the surface, struggling once
more to stay upright. The procedure had not worked.

Back at the aquarium, I went through all of the possible
causes of the dragons' problem and alternate treatments.
After making a few phone calls and checking the literature
again, I had no new ideas. I desperately wanted to save these
special creatures, and not just because of all the time and effort (and money) we'd put into bringing them to Florida.
With their arrival, our aquarium had joined a partnership
known as Project Seahorse, an organization designed to call
attention to the endangered status of sea dragons as well as
sea horses.

Before being shipped halfway across the world, our pair of
dragons had been nurtured and fed in a special setting. We'd
worked with an experienced collector in Australia who holds
one of very few permits issued by the government to collect a limited number of specimens per year. These permits
are given to discourage illegal collecting of adult dragons.
Fishermen catch them not for food but as sources of "alternative" types of human medicine or as souvenir trinkets for
sale in countless numbers of curio stores. It's sad to think of
these animals ending up in such shops. They are so beautiful
in life.

The collector is permitted to collect two types of dragons: one male weedy sea dragon, like the ones we received, and ten male leafy sea dragons. In aquarium lingo, we call them the "weedies" and the "leafies." Sounds a bit like sports teams. The weedies have fewer appendages but tend to be more colorful, with yellows, blues, reds, and lots of decorative white spots. The leafies are the kings of camouflage, with ornate yellow and green fronds that blend in so perfectly with underwater vegetation that they can be hard to spot even when they hover right in front of you.

Like sea horses, sea dragon males carry the eggs, though they are attached to their tails rather than inside pouches, and they can carry up to 250 eggs each. The wild fish are kept in a holding facility until they give birth, and then released back to the wild. When the eggs hatch, the young dragons, only about a quarter of an inch long at birth and practically transparent, are maintained in optimal water conditions, free of predators, and fed several tasty meals a day—sort of an aquatic bed-and-breakfast arrangement. Once they grow to about four inches in length, they are ready to be shipped. This complicated step requires all kinds of permits and paperwork, special containers, and logistical arrangements to ensure the shortest flight routes and times.

—

As a last resort, I decided to aspirate the air directly. Holding a flashlight behind each animal to illuminate the outline of the bladder, I identified suture lines between the bony plates and targeted these with a sharp needle. As a precautionary step, I applied a drop of ophthalmic antibiotic liquid before and after the procedure to help reduce chances of infection. Immediately after the procedure, the fish looked better: both could dive down in the water, if very slowly. I began to hold out a little more hope.

Since the dragons hadn't been eating, we started tube-feeding them mashed-up brine shrimp, hoping to keep their energy levels up. This procedure in itself required creative thinking. We needed to find a tiny flexible tube to place directly into their stomachs while gently holding the fish out of water. I finally found a long catheter, the kind used for spinal taps in humans, that worked perfectly.

A day after the aspiration procedure, they were still alive. We continued to give them antibiotic injections and tube-feeding. Maybe we were finally on the right track. But to my frustration and sorrow, both animals died two days later.

The next step was a painstaking review of our transport procedures. Though we couldn't prove it, my best guess was that the dragons did suffer from supersaturation of their water with oxygen at some point during transport from Australia, possibly during the stopover in Los Angeles, where the animals were repackaged. In preparation for the flight to Tampa, the last leg of their long trip, a fresh supply of oxygen was added to the transport box. Though intended to help, this step may have harmed the precious dragons. We made a number of improvements for the next shipment, including sending one of our biologists to LA to help with the repackaging.

Despite losing both animals, some good things came of this effort. Although the recompression chamber did not save the fish, its use generated a lot of discussion among my veterinary colleagues about alternative treatments as well as about exhibit design. In the long run, this exchange of information increased our collective understanding of sea dragons, including their health care.

More important, the pair of sea dragons in the next shipment arrived in excellent condition; indeed, they thrived, and we were able to open the new exhibit to great reviews. Visitors were fascinated by the creatures' exotic appearance. We have since acquired leafies as well as weedies, and their protection in the wild has improved. These eye-catching fish continue to be among the most popular animals at our aquarium.

ABOUT THE AUTHOR

Though she grew up in the Midwest, Ilze K. Berzins chose to pursue a career in marine biology. She attended Stanford University, earning her BS and MS degrees in biology, and then earned a PhD in zoology from the University of California, Berkeley, with an emphasis on marine invertebrates and behavioral ecology. While assisting with field studies on parasitism in shorebirds, Dr. Berzins became interested in combining aquatic biology with veterinary medicine. She attended veterinary school at the University of California, Davis, and completed an externship at the Minnesota Zoo. After several years in private practice, she enrolled in a three-year fellowship program in comparative pathology at the Johns Hopkins Medical Institutions, and then returned to Minnesota to set up a consulting business in exotic and aquatic animal medicine. For the past ten years, she has served as veterinarian and vice president of biological operations at the Florida Aquarium, where she oversees animal health, husbandry, conservation, research, and dive programs, and is responsible for over fifteen thousand animals, including small mammals, birds, reptiles, and fish. The motto "Leap and the net will appear" has kept her moving forward on an unusual and exciting career path.

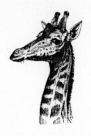

Amali's Example

by Lauren Howard, DVM

Hello. My name is Lauren Howard and I'm calling from the zoo. I was wondering if I could speak with one of your orthopedic surgery instructors? No, I'm not a patient. You see, I have a giraffe with a leg problem. . . ." *Click.* "Hello?"

"Hi, I'm a veterinarian at the Houston Zoo. I have a giraffe with a leg problem and was hoping I could talk to one of your surgical instructors. Yes, I know you don't treat animals. I should try calling the zoo? No, I'm *from* the zoo. . . . Hello?"

Working at a zoo that's next to one of the country's leading medical centers has its advantages. At least that's what I thought when I started calling around looking for advice to help manage my current patient, a young giraffe with a front-leg abnormality. The Texas Medical Center includes two universities and dozens of medical facilities spread out over several blocks across from the zoo. As I dialed medical schools and teaching hospitals, I flipped through a stack of sports-medicine catalogs on my desk, trying to picture a fashionably colored, hinged knee brace fitting onto our patient's scrawny, three-foot-long front leg.

After enduring a variety of on-hold musical selections and repeating myself several times to several medical receptionists, I finally found the contact I was looking for. A human orthopedic surgeon called me back.

"What was this about a giraffe?" he asked kindly.

"Well, she's about four months old. Her hip was dislocated the day she was born, and while she's been recovering from that, she's developing secondary problems in her front legs. I think she needs a support brace for her leg, but nothing we have is working. I've been through dozens of sports-medicine catalogs but I don't think a human brace will fit right. I've got her leg measurements. Do you know of anyone who might be able to make a custom——"

"I've got just the guy for you," he cut me off. "His name is John Fain; let me get you his number."

With one more phone call, I arranged for John to come down to the zoo and join us in our ongoing efforts to get Amali walking normally for the first time in her life.

Born one cool fall morning, Amali did not stand up right away, and her mother accidentally stepped on her, dislocating the calf's right hip. Before the newborn giraffe had a chance to feel the dirt beneath her baby-soft hooves, she found herself in a veterinary specialty hospital. A team of orthopedic surgeons put her leg back in its socket. Lying on the gurney with her head up, Amali surveyed her surroundings as we wheeled her down the halls of the hospital. She seemed to take it all as a matter of course. She had no way of knowing the first few days of life should be any different.

Amali means "charm" in Swahili, a fitting name for this lanky newborn. With her large brown eyes and velvety soft muzzle, our new Masai giraffe calf charmed everyone who met her. Unfortunately, the Hebrew translation of Amali, "result of a long struggle," turned out to be a better description of this spirited little addition to our giraffe family.

After the surgery, the giraffe's hip healed only partially. Because she needed extra support and special care, she was hand-raised on bottles of goat milk. As she grew, Amali could walk but favored her rear leg. As a result, she bore more weight than normal on her front legs, and gradually developed joint problems. Amali's right front leg, in particular, bent out at her knee joint whenever she put weight on it, angling to the side. Because this leg required extra support, we created a makeshift splint using large PVC piping, cut in half and padded with lots of bandaging material. This is a technique used routinely by equine veterinarians for young foals with similar leg deformities. Foals, however, rarely weigh more than 80 pounds and have shorter, more manageable legs. At this point, in early January 2005, Amali weighed about 170 pounds.

Each morning, Amali's keepers (and our largest veterinary technician, Grant, when we could coax him into it) would hold her as still as possible in a corner of the giraffe barn, while they sweated profusely and tried not to let her slip out of their grasp. Often we'd get the padding in place for the PVC splint, only to have our willful giraffe send the gauze and six feet of cotton wrap flying through the air like confetti at a lively New Year's Eve party. To the early morning zoo visitor who happened to catch sight of the strewn bandages through the barn window, it must have looked like quite a fun party indeed. In fact, the procedure was becoming increasingly difficult and even dangerous.

—

"Erica in the clinic to Dr. Lauren. Your specialist is here." Our hospital clerk's voice crackled over my radio. A few minutes later I found John Fain at the zoo clinic, already deep in conversation with a member of our staff, completely at home among the cacophony of smells and sounds common to a zoo hospital. Over the phone a month earlier, John had explained that he was an orthotist and prosthetist, meaning that he designs prosthetic limbs and support braces for his human patients. A self-confessed animal lover and farm boy, John was the perfect fit for our situation. In his standard-issue blue hospital scrubs and shiny white sneakers, he made a cheerful first impression. He'd brought an assistant with him and a shoulder bag of equipment, as well as a digital camera held together with several pieces of duct tape.

At the giraffe barn, I introduced John and his assistant to the keepers and supervisors, who were all eager to help with the creation of the leg mold. The best way to design a well-fitting brace, John had told us, is to make a mold of the leg, which would be used to make a solid model of the leg; then a brace could be made to fit the model. To make the mold, the leg must be placed in a special plaster cast material and held motionless for five to ten minutes while the plaster dries. This is a fairly simple undertaking, I'm sure, when it's performed on cooperative human patients who understand what is being done and why. It's true that John's patients sometimes included small children, as well as residents of the state's prison system who may not always have been completely cooperative. Still, I'm confident that none of his previous patients measured up to Amali.

Now 180 pounds and almost six feet tall, Amali was testing the limits of our staff's ability to restrain her manually. With two people on either side of her and one in front, we pushed her back against a wall of the barn where we could control her a little more easily. It took three more people to extend her right front leg and hold it straight so that John could slide on a protective sleeve, then roll the mold plaster around her leg. Once the mold was in place, we did our best to keep Amali from kicking or bending her leg—or worse, sagging to the ground, as she often did when she realized she was trapped.

Minutes ticked by as we made nervous jokes. The sweat of the people on the top of the Amali-pile trickled down onto the backs and heads of those unlucky enough to be on the bottom. After what seemed an eternity, John snipped the mold off and disappeared into the hazy afternoon with our hard-won prize.

We'd known all along that we could not reverse the source of the problem—the damage in Amali's right hip. Even at the tender age of five months she was too heavy to undergo another hip surgery or hip replacement. Instead, we'd focused on the things we could fix: her front legs and right knee. By protecting these joints, we could give Amali a chance to walk without pain. Masai giraffes can grow up to fourteen feet and weigh 1,200 pounds. It was hard to imagine our little patient ever reaching this size; yet, if she did, the stress on her damaged hip would be severe.

A week after our strenuous efforts to create Amali's leg mold, John came back to the zoo to show us the result. I still had not quite gotten the kink out of my neck or the sawdust out of my boots when I was once again escorting John and his assistant to the giraffe barn. From the wariness with which the keepers and supervisors watched us enter, I guessed I was not the only one still suffering from the effects of our last wrestling match with Amali.

John put his bag down and fished around inside it, pulling out Amali's first brace with a flourish. Made of shiny white plastic with animal cartoons stenciled on it in bright primary colors, the brace looked more suited to a child's bedroom than to our musty giraffe barn. It was split along the sides into two long halves, and was to be held in place by four bright white Velcro straps. On the inside, the brace was padded with a soft white foam to prevent rubbing, and it still smelled vaguely of glue.

From the grins on the faces in the giraffe barn, the brace was clearly a hit among the staff. But what would Amali think? Would we have to wrestle her to put it on? She was standing nonchalantly by herself in a sunny section of the giraffe yard. When she saw us coming, she started drooling, anticipating the bottle that was sure to come (and would provide a necessary distraction). While she sucked on the bottle, John and I gently placed the brace around her front leg and fastened the straps. It fit perfectly, extending from just below her elbow to just above her ankle. When Amali finished her bottle, she nosed my blond ponytail as I bent over her to help John with the fitting. Soon I felt warm giraffe saliva sliding down my neck. Amali had developed a taste for certain fruity shampoos, and often sucked on my hair as eagerly as she did her bottle.

Holding our breaths, we stepped back to watch her in her new brace. She took a tentative step forward, bore full weight on the leg, and started to walk carefully around the yard. Clearly her little giraffe brain knew there was something different about her leg. Soon she decided this new thing attached to her wasn't such a big deal. After all, it was a nice, sunny day—and hey, aren't those yams you're holding?

Reaching up to hand Amali a thin slice of yam, I silently congratulated my patient—the first giraffe in Texas to have her own custom-made leg brace. Then I thanked John, who had generously donated his time, that of his assistants, and all of the materials for the brace. Grateful handshakes and the occasional soggy giraffe kiss were all he required for services rendered.

Thanks to the design of the brace and Amali's enthusiasm for her bottles, we never had to restrain her in order to put the brace on or take it off. With the leg straight and protected from further damage, the next step was exercise and rehabilitation, a challenge taken up by Dr. Mark Haugland, a local equine surgeon. He had years of experience treating horses with leg problems very similar to Amali's. I knew the basic principles of managing limb issues in hoofed animals ("If it's straight, make it bend; if it's bent, make it straight"), but the nuances of treating an angular versus a flexural deformity were beyond me.

Dr. Mark had an affable bedside manner and was remarkably enthusiastic about examining a patient we couldn't restrain and that he might not even be able to touch. Over several visits to the giraffe barn, he helped us define Amali's multiple orthopedic problems and focus on improving the health of her front legs and her right knee. On his recommendation, we slowly increased the length of time Amali was in the brace until she was wearing it twenty hours a day and could lie down and sleep comfortably in it. He also recommended daily physical therapy for all of her limbs, which the keepers performed religiously and without complaint.

Before long, the shiny plastic exterior of the brace was scuffed and scratched, the white Velcro straps had darkened to an earthy brown, and the pristine padding on the inside had begun smelling like a sweaty giraffe leg. John Fain and his assistants made four more braces for Amali as she grew taller and taller.

Amali's physical therapy sessions and colorful leg brace attracted the attention of our zoo visitors. We'd anticipated their questions ("What happened? Is it broken? Does it hurt?") and posted signs around her exhibit explaining why the baby giraffe was wearing a brace. The response was overwhelming. Visitors not only expressed empathy and support for our efforts, they also shared accounts of people in their own lives who needed special braces or had lost a limb. Some told their stories directly to zoo staff; others called or sent e-mail.

One story about a little girl named Michaela touched us all. Her mother, Denise, wrote to us asking for a photograph of Amali in her brace. Michaela had suffered a hand injury when she was a premature infant. Despite multiple surgeries, she'd worn a brace on her wrist ever since. Now a willful four-year-old, Michaela had begun resisting wearing her brace, particularly at preschool and in front of her peers.

During a recent visit to the zoo, mother and daughter had turned a corner and found Amali standing nearby. The giraffe was contentedly wearing her newest brace, this one covered with purple butterflies (John felt she'd outgrown the brightly colored baby animals). Michaela had found a friend—and a role model. We happily sent Denise the photo, and learned that Michaela had carried it to school and shared it with her friends; more than that, she'd resumed wearing her own brace without complaint or argument. Denise described her daughter's transformation as immediate—and remarkable, as if a lightbulb had suddenly been turned on.

Moved by Denise's story, we invited Michaela back to the zoo to meet Amali in person. Normally full of energy, with bouncing blond curls and an insatiable curiosity, Michaela grew uncharacteristically shy and perhaps a little fearful as she gazed up at her four-legged inspiration. But fear soon turned to adoration when Amali bent her long neck over Michaela's head to reach for a piece of carrot in the keeper's hand. The little girl giggled at the giraffe's long scratchy tongue and her tendency to drool all over her visitors.

Denise had to visit five different orthopedic offices before she found one that carried John's purple butterfly print, but the effort was well worth it. When Michaela learned her next brace would look like Amali's, she actually became enthusiastic about her next fitting.

To our amazement, Amali's front legs straightened out over the next several months. The giraffe weaned herself off the bottle and then began to grow quickly. By the age of eleven months, she no longer needed the brace.

Then came a devastating shock: we arrived at work one late summer morning to find our young giraffe dead. She had fractured her neck against a barn wall and died instantly. We could only assume that her clumsy gait and bad hip had contributed to the accident. Something might have startled her and caused her to trip. We reminded ourselves that Amali faced an uncertain quality of life as an adult giraffe—that her hip and knee could have caused significant long-term problems. Even so, we were not prepared to say good-bye so suddenly, so unexpectedly.

The entire zoo community mourned the loss of our brave little giraffe. Each of us took solace in what we had learned from Amali. Her keepers had experienced firsthand the rewards of training and conditioning a young giraffe; their work had made a tremendous difference in our ability to care for Amali. I learned that if you are persistent enough, you can find the help you need, even in unlikely places: people will pitch in and help. And we all learned from Michaela. Her relationship with Amali showed us how much animals can help children adjust to difficult situations.

Our zoo's struggle to treat a young animal with a crippling condition had an impact far beyond its gates. Amali touched the entire community. We now have a formal relationship with a local children's orthopedic hospital, and the giraffe barn is always one of their favorite stops.

Even two years after Amali's death, Michaela remembers the sensation of Amali's sticky tongue on her fingers and how it felt to be the only child in her kindergarten class who had a giraffe for a friend. She will soon undergo a surgery to lengthen and straighten her arm. Though Denise knows the procedure won't be easy, she also knows her daughter will take it all in stride, including the months of physical therapy ahead. Now a spirited, confident six-year-old, Michaela recently announced that she might want to be a zoo veterinarian when she grows up.

ABOUT THE AUTHOR

Lauren L. Howard grew up in Maryland with a houseful of pet rodents. She became interested in zoo medicine during high school, thanks to her father, a biomedical engineer, and his acquaintance with veterinarians at the National Zoo in Washington, DC. She received her veterinary degree from the Virginia–Maryland Regional College of Veterinary Medicine in southwestern Virginia and then spent a year as small animal medicine and surgery intern at the Oradell Animal Hospital in New Jersey. She completed a residency in zoo medicine in a joint program between the University of California, Davis, and the Zoological Society of San Diego. While in San Diego, Dr. Howard participated in the

California condor reintroduction project in Baja California, Mexico. A staff veterinarian at the Houston Zoo since 2005, she lives south of Houston with her husband, Doug, a small animal veterinarian, and their two dogs, three cats, and J.C., their pet lizard—a bearded dragon.

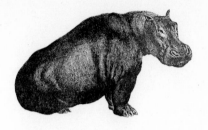

Alfredito the Hippo

by Susan Mikota, DVM

Michael and I looked excitedly at each other as the flight attendant announced the final approach to San Salvador. I stared at the photograph of Alfredito clutched in my hand, focusing on the image of the broken tooth we had come to repair.

"Are you ready?" I asked Michael.

"Sure," he said confidently.

I wished I didn't feel so nervous. It seemed like only yesterday that I had received a letter from my friend and colleague, Dr. Carlos Suazo, who had participated in our veterinary study program at the Audubon Zoo in New Orleans.

> *Dear Dr. Mikota,*
>
> *We have a serious problem on our hands. Our hippopotamus, a sixteen-year-old three-thousand pound male*

(fondly known to the public as "Don Hipo" or "Alfredito"),
shows an eight-inch-deep vertical cavity in his large
right incisor. We are at a loss to know how to sedate the
animal or to perform the necessary procedure. Can you
help?

Dr. Carlos Suazo, National Zoo, El Salvador

From the picture Dr. Suazo sent, it was clear Alfredito had broken his lower right tusk near the gum line, exposing the nerve and blood vessels at the center of the tooth. In other words, he had an open root canal. The open cavity had begun to fill with food material, and Dr. Suazo feared the tooth would become infected. Alfredito's behavior had changed. He seemed dull and quiet, both possible signs of pain.

I discussed the case with Michael McCullar, our zoo's dental technician. We decided that Alfredito needed a root canal procedure and began making plans. The project would present quite a challenge. Despite many calls to colleagues, I could not find anyone who had done a root canal on a hippo; they all agreed it would be a risky procedure. Michael would need to make special instruments. We knew we'd need to take a variety of equipment, including our dart gun. We also knew we might encounter tanks and even gunfire in the streets of San Salvador: in 1991, the country was in the midst of political turmoil. We agreed that while we couldn't do much to prepare for the unknown, we could do our best to plan everything else, right down to the last dental pick.

Although I had been to Central America several times to teach in zoo veterinary workshops, this was the first time I'd be carrying darting equipment on such a trip. I wanted to

make sure we followed every procedure properly so that
things would proceed without a hitch. I consulted the El
Salvador embassy to see if I would need any special permits
for the dart gun. I asked the airline staff the same questions,
explaining that at first glance the gun resembles an ordinary
rifle. We would also be carrying potent narcotics to use for
sedation. I found out we'd need special permits and packing
to transport the carbon dioxide cartridges that are used to
power the dart gun. We requested and received these permits, as well as a letter from the embassy approving a dona-
tion of medications.

Having never been to El Salvador, Michael and I were
uncertain what supplies would be available. We decided to
bring everything we needed: syringes, needles, fluids, IV
sets, antibiotics, and, of course, emergency drugs . . . just in
case. Our supplies filled two big trunks. Our dart gun was in
its own special case.

—

As we retrieved our baggage at the San Salvador airport, I
looked anxiously around for Dr. Suazo. He was nowhere to
be seen. We stalled for as long as possible and then proceeded
through customs. I had hoped Dr. Suazo would be there to
escort us through the process so that he could explain the
equipment we were bringing into the country. As I placed the
dart gun case on the table, the customs inspector asked, *"¿Que
es esto?"* (What is this?)

I froze for a second as my brain struggled to convert from
English to Spanish. *"Es un rifle,"* I responded. His eyes got big
as he opened the case and picked up the dart rifle. *"Este rifle es*

para animales," I said quickly. *"Para anesthesia."* He glared at me as he turned the rifle over and then began to take it apart. I was getting more nervous. I glanced at Michael. He looked worried. *"Por favor, señor—este es importante—estés es para ayudar Alfredito, el hipo."* ("Please, sir—this is important—it is to help Alfredito, the hippo.")

The customs official stopped and looked up, smiling broadly. *"Ah, Alfredito—muy bueno—me gusto mucho—por favor pasar. ¡Buena suerte!"* ("Ah, Alfredito—very good—I like him very much—please go on. Good luck!")

With great relief, we walked into the terminal. As we passed through the door, zoo officials, TV cameras, and a horde of children greeted us. Guillermo Saade, an eight-year-old boy, presented me with a dozen yellow roses from the children of San Salvador. Another child handed me a newspaper. On the front page was a story about the two Americans who were coming to save Alfredito. The story on the opposite side of the page was an article about the president of El Salvador. His name was also Alfredito. Speechless, I nodded my thanks. All I could think was "What if I lose this hippo?"

It was not an unreasonable fear. Hippos are notoriously difficult to anesthetize safely, even under ideal conditions. For one thing, it is important that a hippo land on its sternum when it falls from the effects of the drug. If it ends up on an incline with its head lower than the rest of its body, there is a possibility of excessive pressure on the diaphragm, which can result in suffocation. A hippo's large size makes it difficult—if not impossible—to reposition it under anesthesia. And hippos lack accessible veins, which can be a real problem in an emergency when IV drugs can be lifesaving.

As our driver navigated the streets of San Salvador, the reality of the situation hit me. Here we were, in a foreign country, full of political strife, getting ready to immobilize their only hippo, an animal that was obviously beloved by all. Though I tried not to notice, there were indeed huge green army-style tanks at almost every corner. We passed many damaged buildings riddled with bullet holes. We frequently heard gunfire. Our hosts were apparently used to this sound: they didn't jump as I did every time it occurred.

The next day I came to understand why Alfredito was such a star. Children and adults crowded around his exhibit to watch while his keeper placed whole heads of lettuce and cabbage in Alfredito's huge, open mouth. This species can be quite temperamental and dangerous. I'd never seen a keeper go into an exhibit with a hippo. But Alfredito and his keeper both seemed quite relaxed. So Michael and I went into the exhibit with them.

While the keeper scratched the hippo's chin, we were able to get a close look at the broken tooth. We stood right next to our patient and watched him eat a few more heads of cabbage. Although Alfredito was eager for the treats, it was clear he was in pain. The keeper was careful to place the offerings on the good side of his mouth. Watching them, I too became enraptured by Alfredito. He was adorable—and quite the showman. He seemed to enjoy the attention. It was clear why he had so many admirers. Now I was one of them, and tomorrow his life would be in my hands.

We met with Dr. Suazo and the zoo staff that afternoon to plan the procedure for the next morning. Alfredito would need to be fasted, a routine step for any large herbivore, as they sometimes regurgitate while under the effects of anesthesia. The sloped entrance to the pool was also particularly dangerous. If the hippo succumbed to the effects of the anesthetic while attempting to get back into his pool, he would go down with his head below the rest of his body. In such a position, the sheer weight of his abdominal organs pushing up against his diaphragm could cause his lungs to collapse. We would need to drain his pool and build a fence around it. We would also start early to avoid the hot sun, which could cause Alfredito to overheat. Dr. Suazo translated as we discussed the procedure and our requirements.

The procedure began at seven the next morning. I carefully loaded the narcotic anesthetic, known by its trade name M99, into the dart, then loaded the dart into the rifle. I walked slowly up to Alfredito and fired. The dart hit the back of his right thigh, but the needle bounced. It was impossible to know if he had received the full dose. Hippo skin is very thick and difficult to puncture. If the dart does not hit exactly perpendicular, it will do what this one did: bounce. We watched Alfredito, waiting to see signs of the anesthetic taking effect, but nothing seemed to be happening. Alfredito lumbered slowly around his exhibit and, after an hour, it was clear that although he was sedated, he wasn't ready to go to sleep.

I loaded another dart with great care. M99 is a very good drug but quite dangerous to handle: as little as one-tenth of a milliliter can be fatal to humans. I fired the dart, and this time it stuck. But Alfredito continued to amble around, and after twenty minutes, we decided the M99 had not injected. The needle I'd used had a large diameter opening, or bore. It must have been blocked by a small skin plug, just enough to prevent the drug from injecting. By this time, it was beginning to get hot; I instructed the zoo staff to prepare a tent to place over Alfredito to protect him from the hot sun. With the tent in place, the third time turned out to be the charm. Alfredito finally succumbed to the effects of my next dart.

Luckily, the hippo went down in a good position on his sternum and near the back of his exhibit, away from the gathering crowd. Michael jumped into action and began cleaning and preparing the tooth while I monitored Alfredito's respiration and heartbeat. About fifteen minutes into the procedure, the hippo's breathing began to slow. Then it abruptly stopped. I held my breath and for a brief second I felt my own heart stop. *Oh no,* I thought, *I cannot let this animal die.*

With the narcotic reversal agent in hand—the only option I could think of at that point—I searched unsuccessfully for a vein. Almost simultaneously, Dr. Suazo handed me a syringe of doxapram, a respiratory stimulant, and said, "In his tongue." *Good idea,* I thought. I quickly injected the doxapram and leapt over the sleeping Alfredito to search for a vein on the other side of his body. Luckily, I found one and was able to inject the reversal agent into Alfredito's vein while the adrenaline rushed through my own. The silence of the crowd of zoo staff and visitors hugging Alfredito's exhibit added to the tension. Suddenly a cheer arose: Alfredito had taken a long, deep breath.

While all of this was going on, Michael had continued to work on the tooth and miraculously had managed to finish the procedure before the full effects of the anesthesia were reversed. We gave Alfredito his antibiotic injection and then Guillermo, the child who'd handed me the flowers, was allowed a special close-up visit. With cameras flashing all around us, I assured him that his favorite animal was going to be all right.

But our worries were not over. Difficult anesthetic procedures can predispose to a serious condition called capture myopathy, a painful muscle problem that can be fatal. It is caused by the pressure on the downside muscles produced by the hippo's weight while it sleeps under anesthesia combined with changes in blood flow and blood pressure produced by the drug.

For the next twenty-four hours, we observed Alfredito for any adverse signs.

To our huge relief, everything seemed okay. The next day there was a picture of Michael and me on the front page of the newspaper, accompanied by a very long story of what had transpired. The reporter had written about Alfredito in detail, with dramatic descriptions of the action, so that the story read more like a novel than a news report. We were quite impressed.

When we returned to the zoo to check on our patient, the hippo seemed to be back to his old self. Children crowded around his exhibit, watching joyfully as Alfredito chomped down on whole heads of lettuce and cabbage—pain-free.

Three months later, we were invited back to the zoo to re-examine Alfredito. Our patient was doing fine, so they put us to work. Over the course of three days, we anesthetized and treated a grizzly bear, a lion, and four leopards. Michael performed seventeen root canals!

ABOUT THE AUTHOR

Susan K. Mikota's career in wildlife medicine began the year she graduated from the University of Illinois College of Veterinary Medicine. She says, "I was simply in the right place at the right time when the Audubon Zoo in New Orleans was transitioning into a world-class zoo. I'd had only two weeks of on-the-job training when attending veterinarian Dr. Andy Gutter was offered a trip to Africa. He left me the phone numbers of two other zoo veterinarians and gave me these instructions: 'Don't kill the gorilla.' Luckily, the gorilla and I both survived." In 1985, Dr. Mikota became the zoo's first full-time veterinarian. In subsequent years, she has served as president of the Association of Avian Veterinarians, chairperson of the Zoo Conservation Outreach Group, director of veterinary services at Audubon Zoo, director of veterinary research and animal health for the Audubon Center for Research of Endangered Species (ACRES), and chair of the National Tuberculosis Working Group for Zoo and Wildlife Species. Dr. Mikota is currently director of veterinary programs and research for Elephant Care International, a nonprofit organization she cofounded.

A Final Word

Few of us thought about cancer therapy, vaccinations, or intensive care for free-living wild animals until their numbers began to plummet. Even ten years ago, most zoo vets could easily distinguish in their minds what was appropriate care for a wild animal living in captivity versus one living in its natural habitat. Vets who worked in aquaria treated only the aquatic animals within their own and similar facilities. The title "wildlife vet" signified someone who worked exclusively with free-living wild animals. As we pointed out in the introduction to this book, the distinction is less important now.

There are only so many poison dart frogs, saltwater crocodiles, giant pandas, sea dragons, beluga whales, and mountain gorillas left on earth. Populations of lions, tigers, bears, and many other species that could once withstand a disease outbreak or natural disaster now need our help. The health of each individual wild animal matters, whether it's free-living or captive.

As natural habitats are damaged or destroyed, the words "endangered species" have become a household phrase. Even in remote places, wild animals are exposed to polluted air, water, and soil. They also face a higher risk of disease because of increased contact with people and domestic animals. Most, if not all, of these changes are the result of human activity.

Modern zoos, aquaria, and wildlife parks now invest in conservation programs, and many have updated their exhibits and education programs to reflect the importance of protecting entire ecosystems. Protected areas and national parks are also hiring more vets to monitor the health of rare species and intervene by treating individual animals when necessary.

In the course of our careers, we zoo vets now have the opportunity to practice medicine in a variety of settings. We possess a unique set of skills that allows us to treat the individual animal while also considering the population as a whole. We know how to explain the science behind the medicine, and why some medical decisions are more problematic than others. Our challenge is to take these efforts one step further.

On a world scale, the health of all living things is connected. From a holistic point of view, a wild animal can remain healthy only if the humans and other animals in its ecosystem are also healthy. The negative corollary is that there's a chain reaction when something goes wrong.

Even the king of the jungle, the African lion, has succumbed to diseases like dog distemper, an infection spread by village dogs in the Serengeti to free-ranging jackals and wild dogs. The lions were infected secondarily. In the suburbs of Los Angeles, raccoons picked up distemper from feral dogs, as they often do, and spread it to a wildlife sanctuary, where it killed lions and other big cats.

A similar domino effect continues to affect sea otters off the coast of California. Every year several die from a brain infection caused by a parasite that originates in two species, the feral cat and the Virginia opossum. Soil erosion and clogged tributaries contribute to excess runoff of rainwater that flows into the ocean, carrying with it the scat of these animals. Once in the food chain of kelp and abalone, the disease can be picked up by the sea otters—and potentially by seafood-loving humans as well.

Zoo vets have begun playing an active role in restoring the balance of nature, though the workload ahead seems to stretch to infinity. In cooperation with other scientists, we have managed in recent years to restore a handful of endangered species to the wild. Clearly, the chain reaction of ill health can be reversed if we work together. By taking advantage of the fact that everything *is* connected, zoo vets can make a positive difference.

When a doctor heals a patient, human or animal, the entire ecosystem benefits. When public health officials eradicate measles and polio, the world will become a healthier place for wild animals too. Health professionals, decisionmakers, and ordinary citizens can set policies that protect existing healthy ecosystems and target those that need our help. If we act quickly, wisely, and collaboratively, we can even contain emerging diseases.

It's essential that vets who work with wild animals find ways to integrate their expertise into the broad scheme of things. We need to share what we know and how we feel about wild animals and their health, and do our best to promote healthy ecosystems in the places where we work. The stories in this book reflect the willingness within our profession to do just that—to talk to people as well as animals.

Lucy H. Spelman, DVM

Acknowledgments

We thank our contributing authors for their enthusiastic participation in this project from the beginning, as well as the many veterinarians who directly or indirectly contributed their expertise to help the wild animal patients in each story. In other words, we thank all vets who work with wild animals!

We are also grateful to keepers, animal caretakers, biologists, trackers, and rangers—paid and volunteer—for their tireless efforts on behalf of the animals under their care.

We thank Jody Rein, our literary agent, for her support, encouragement, constructive criticism, expertise, timely advice, and fascination with wild animals. Without Jody, this book would still be a good idea in the backs of our minds, and we would never have found Danielle Perez, our equally terrific editor at Bantam Dell.

For their encouragement, we are grateful to our many friends and colleagues. Special thanks go to: Bill Adler, Clark Bunting, Alan Cutler, Jackie Jeffers, Jo Gayle Howard, Franchon Smithson, Diane McTurk, Roy Mashima, Julie Mashima, Athena Mylonas, Jennie Rice, Trish Silber, and Mary Tanner.

About the Authors

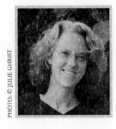

LUCY H. SPELMAN, DVM, is the regional veterinary manager for the Mountain Gorilla Veterinary Project in central Africa, based in Rwanda. She is the former director of the Smithsonian National Zoo in Washington, D.C., and has been featured on Animal Planet and the Discovery Channel.

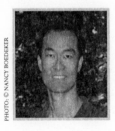

TED Y. MASHIMA, DVM, is director of academic and research affairs for the Association of American Veterinary Medical Colleges, based in Washington, D.C.